SILVER DENTAL FILLINGS

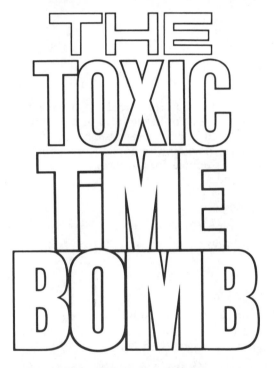

CAN THE MERCURY IN YOUR DENTAL FILLINGS POISON YOU?

SAM Z

D1530869

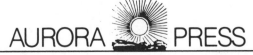

AURORA PRESS

P.O. Box 573   Santa Fe, N.M. 87504

First published in 1984
Second Revised Edition 1986
Third Expanded Edition 1994
Aurora Press, Inc.
P.O. Box 573
Santa Fe, N.M. 87504
Printed in the United States of America
ISBN: 0-943358-22-1
Library of Congress Catalogue Card No:
84-072253

DEDICATION

To my wife Helen who supported me so unselfishly during the researching and writing of this book and whose primary reward was to become a temporary "mercury widow." To my son Michael whose intense interest in the subject convinced me to assist him in doing research on the potential toxicity of mercury and dental amalgam and to his wife Peggy who so ably assisted in editing the final manuscript.

To that small group of dentists, other health care providers and researchers who in the face of overwhelming peer and establishment pressures continued their individual efforts to prove the potential toxicity of dental amalgam fillings. Their motivating force has always been the health and well being of the patient.

Most of all this book is dedicated to the millions of people who are unaware that their "Silver Dental Fillings" actually contain more mercury than silver and that the mercury escaping from their silver fillings has the potential of seriously affecting their health.

TABLE OF CONTENTS

FOREWORD
By Jeffrey Bland, Ph.D.

The field of dental amalgam and its relationship to chronic mercurial immunosuppressive disorders has recently been revived and has received considerable attention. For years it has been assumed that once amalgam restorative work is in place it becomes fixed and does not liberate mercury to systemic circulation. However, recent information seems to indicate that there are a number of variables which may contribute to increased ablation of mercury amalgams, including galvanic currents, plaque and pH of the oral cavity. Given these observations there is concern that in individuals who undergo more rapid amalgam ablation there may be enhanced accumulation of systemic mercury which could have significant influences upon the immune system through lymphocyte inactivity or alteration of T/suppressor/helper ratios. The recent work of Eggleston seems to indicate that there is a relationship between immunosuppressive effects and mercury amalgams in some patients. Given this, the book "Silver Dental Fillings: The Toxic Time Bomb" comes at a very appropriate time. It alerts the reader to the need for more research and understanding of the role that mercury amalgam may have on chronic health dysfunction. It appears that the position of many dental researchers has been that mercury is safe in the mouth as applied and does not require extensive additional research. This book seems to open the question for reevaluation and exploration and it appears that, at least for those who are mercury-sensitive and who have more rapid ablation of mercury amalgams, this message may have considerable importance in terms of their long-term health. I believe this book is going to contribute to an enlightenment in the general field and to more extensive research which is needed to compare the safety of amalgam restorative work to other alternatives such as precious metals and plastics.

Jeffrey Bland, Ph.D.
Director
Laboratory for Nutritional
Supplement Analysis
Linus Pauling Institute of
Science and Medicine

INTRODUCTION

The greatest health controversy of our time is brewing. The issue of this controversy is whether the human body accommodates, without lasting ill effects, to its exposure to the metal mercury. Mercury is utilized in the practice of dentistry, medicine, manufacture of pharmaceutical and cosmetic preparations, industry, in agricultural applications as fungicides/pesticides, and the environmental contamination resulting from some of the applications mentioned. The final insult to our bodies being the actual consumption of mercury that has become a part of the food chain.

If our bodies do not accommodate adequately, does this mean that our exposures to mercury and other toxic metals may in fact be causing untold damage that in some instances may even be irreparable? Can it be possible that mercury may be the "key", the single factor responsible for so many unexplainable health problems experienced by man, which are of unknown origin or etiology?

It is not my intent in writing this book to address all the possible sources of mercury contamination of the human body. This book will address only its use in dentistry, which I consider to be the central issue to the overall problem of human exposure.

Simply stated, the issue is whether the standard filling material utilized by the dental profession world-wide since its invention in the year 1819 is safe.

The material in question is called amalgam and takes several forms or compositions. It is most commonly referred to as silver amalgam or just silver. The material is provided to the dentist as two separate entities which he or his staff must then mix together. The final product is then placed into the tooth cavity to fill or reconstruct the tooth. The first entity of amalgam is an alloy or mixture of the following metals: not less than 65% silver; not less than 25% tin; not more than 6% copper; and not more than 2% zinc. The second entity of amalgam is pure elemental mercury. The two components are then mixed together in a 50–50 ratio so that the end product utilized by the dentist to reconstruct your tooth is approximately 50% mercury.

There are two basic questions related to the use of amalgam. The first deals with a scientific phenomenon that results in the generation of an electrical current when two dissimilar metals are immersed or enveloped by an electrolyte fluid. In this case your saliva fulfills the role of an electrolyte and the amalgam provides dissimilar metals. Is there an electrical current being continually generated in our mouths because of this and, if so, is it causing any problems or damage? The second question is whether once the amalgam is installed in the tooth, does the material remain "locked" inside the tooth or does some of the metal escape from the tooth, in some fashion, and enter our bodies?

If some form of the involved metals does come out of the filling material and enter the body, does it cause any harm? Bearing in mind that silver, mercury, tin, and even copper can all be highly toxic to the human body systems, this book will attempt to provide you with the facts based on existing published research, so that you can make the final judgement.

Is the controversy worth reading about? Regardless of how you may ultimately judge the facts, the answer is an unqualified YES! Here is why. Those individuals that claim that the metals in the amalgam do come out and do enter the body, also claim that the following health related problems can be caused as a direct result:

BLEEDING GUMS
INCREASED SALIVATION
SOUR-METALLIC TASTE
FACIAL PARALYSIS
IRREGULAR HEARTBEAT
DEPRESSION
STRONG PAINS IN THE LEFT PART OF CHEST
RETINAL BLEEDING
DIM VISION
UNCONTROLLABLE EYE MOVEMENT
IRRITABILITY
VERTIGO
HEADACHES
JOINT PAINS
PAINS IN LOWER BACK
ETC. ETC. ETC. ETC.

Do you have any amalgam fillings in your mouth? (I estimate about 85% of the population in the United States has one or more amalgam fillings in their mouth). Have you experienced any of the above symptoms or signs? Is your interest piqued? Are you interested in your personal health and well being? Then, please read on, as the facts get much more interesting.

Sam Ziff retired from the U.S. Air Force, with the rank of Lt. Colonel, in 1970. He is the publisher of *The Bioprobe*, which provides in depth reviews of pertinent scientific literature, regarding mercury amalgam toxicity.

He has extensively researched the potential toxicity of mercury and dental amalgam. Through his publication, he has acted as an "International Clearinghouse", by networking, gathering the most current information available and making it available to both professionals and the general public. He currently resides in Florida with his wife Helen.

CHAPTER 1

MERCURY IN MEDICINE AND DENTISTRY

Heavy metals are defined as those with the greatest atomic weights. If you haven't had chemistry that statement won't mean much to you. For our purposes, just say they are heavier than most other minerals and none have been identified as being essential to life.

The soil and water on this planet have always had some natural concentration of these metals and as a result, man has always had some exposure to them. Mineral content of soils varies greatly in different regions and, as a consquence, the first poisonings probably occurred in those areas where there was a high concentration of the heavy metals, resulting in toxic metallic contamination of the food and water supply.

Man, in his never ending struggle to improve his quality of life, has increased the metallic contamination of his environment to the point where it is the major source of heavy metal pollution and poisoning. Metals even leach out of our cookware and eating utensils. In fact, cast iron cookware used to be the major source of iron in our diets. We use constituents of these toxic heavy metals for a myriad of purposes ranging from medicines as thereapeutic agents to fungicides and pesticides that we spray on the crops we grow and eat and the tobacco we may smoke.

If that wasn't sufficient, we polluted our environment with lead by the addition of tetraethyl-lead to our gasoline and burned fossil fuels like coal that contained many heavy metals including mercury. Yes, I am sure that very few of us ever realized that those huge coal-burning utility plants spew hundreds of tons of mercury out of their smoke stacks every year, year in and year out. The same is true for all the homes and factories that still burn coal.

Man in his infinite wisdom has always been capable of doing things in the name of "progress" without due regard to the impact and effect his acts or creations have on life in later years or generations of the species.

Such is truly the situation in the case of mercury utilized in medicine and dentistry. Although my concern is primarily with amalgam and dentistry, a section on the history of mercury in medicine is included just to keep everything in perspective.

I.
THE HISTORY OF MERCURY IN MEDICINE

The use of mercury in medicine predates its use in dentistry by centuries. As early as 500 B.C. there is evidence that India was using mercury as a drug. However, it appears that it was the Arabian physicians who first studied the use of mercury as a drug and introduced the use of a mercurial ointment in the 10th century.

Mercurial therapy made its way into Europe around the 13th century and spread throughout Europe. It was not widely prescribed until the 16th century. It was during this period that mercury ointments became "the drug of choice" in the treatment of syphilis. It was also in the 16th century that the controversy over the use of mercury came into focus. It was identified as the cause of poisoning among miners working in the mercury mines of Austria and Spain. The symptomatology of mercury poisoning was described as: tremor (shivering without feeling cold), gastrointestinal disturbances, oral infections, and blackening of teeth.

During the 17th century, again because of trembling, paralysis, malnutrition and premature deaths among mercury mine workers, the first standards for occupational health were introduced—the workday for mercury miners was reduced from 16 hours to 6 hours. It was also at this time that medical use of mercury seemed to fall from favor. Mercury and other metals were identified as occupational hazards for miners, gilders, chemists, potters, tinsmiths, glassworkers, mirror makers, painters, and medical personnel. There was even a law suit brought against the owner of a chemical factory that was manufacturing mercury chloride. The charge was the pollution of the local environment which contributed to an increased death rate in the neighborhood. What is really significant about this incident is that it happened in 1713 and it was one of the first public outcrys over continued use of mercury with its many adverse effects against health. Towards the end of the 17th century two important events occurred: Mercury was identified as a neurotoxicant and, in 1685, mercury nitrate began to be used in France in the preparation of fur felt, to be utilized in the making of hats.

In the 18th century, continued use of mercury therapy sparked many major controversies, especially in England. The proponents for and against took to the press to convey their positions. Regardless of the position taken, whether you were an advocate or a critic, mercury was an important topic of interest for 18th century practitioners. It was towards the end of the 18th century that the practice of prescribing mercury found its way into medical practice in the United States. Right from the outset there was controversy, intense enemies on its use as well as ardent and convinced supporters.

It was during the 19th century, that scientific experimentation with mercury began. In fact, one of the first reports on mercury's fetotoxic effects resulted from an experiment performed by Gaspard, in which he exposed fly eggs to mercury vapor in inadequate conditions of temperature and humidity. In the experimental group, no eggs hatched, whereas in the control group (not exposed to mercury vapor) hundreds of eggs hatched.

The belief that mercury cured venereal disease engendered a generalized false belief among most physicians that if mercury could cure venereal disease it could also cure other diseases that were not curable with other medicines. As a result of this false perception of mercury's efficacy its use increased dramatically during the 19th century. It became the drug of choice for almost any problem from chronic diarrhea to typhoid fever. It was also during this time that use of mercury as a diuretic agent became established as acceptable clinical practice.

Organomercurials retained their place in the modern pharmacopeia, even after several deaths as a direct result of their use and even after the introduction of other diuretics (thiazides) that did not have the toxicity of mercurials.

In the last quarter of the 19th century, French scientists discovered that mercurials possessed germicidal and antiseptic capabilities and introduced their use into clinical practice. Although side effects and deaths were reported shortly after it was introduced as an antiseptic, that didn't stop its use. In fact, a hundred years later, in 1984 you can still obtain mercurial antiseptics over the counter. The availability of pharmaceutical preparations may change in the not too distant future as the FDA is proposing the ban of all over the counter products made with mercury. This action is finally being proposed because a child recently died from using merthiolate (prescribed by her physician) to treat an infection in her ear.

During the 20th century industrial and agricultural use of mercury compounds reached their peak. There have also been some of the more severe human tragedies in the world as a result. Poisoning from mercury has caused the deaths of thousands of innocent unsuspecting people. The major incidents occurred at Minamata Bay, Japan; Northern Iraq; Guatemala; Ghana; Almagordo, New Mexico. More recently, during 1983, there were eight different incidents of Kawasaki-type disease reported from different areas of the United States to the Center for Disease Control (CDC) in Atlanta. (CDC has not concluded that mercury is the causative agent in Kawasaki disease).

The major incidents of widespread poisoning were the catalyst for focusing world-wide attention of the scientific community on the highly toxic nature of mercury and demonstrated graphically the disastrous results of human ignorance and industrial carelessness. Because of their importance to us all in understanding the insidious nature of this substance, I am going to relate in more detail some of these major incidents.

The first two incidents took place in Japan, during the period of 1953–1965. The first epidemic at Minamata Bay identified methyl mercury as the environmental contaminant involved. The second epidemic occurred in the Agano River in Niigata. In Minamata, 121 people were identified as being poisoned by methylmercury and of this number, 46 subsequently died from the poison. In Niigata there were 6 deaths out of a total of 47 cases identified as having methyl mercury poisoning. In both Minamata and Niigata the researchers were finally able to establish a relationship between the disease and the amount of fish consumed. The source of contamination to the fish was identified as the discharges from factories using mercuric chloride catalysts in the manufacture of vinyl chloride and acetaldehyde. Individuals consuming the contaminated fish suffered a generalized degenerative neurological disease. The researchers also clearly established that the mercury was penetrating the placental membrane in pregnant women and affecting the fetus. In fact the name of "Fetal Minamata Disease" was used to identify fetuses poisoned by methyl mercury because 6% of the births in Minamata resulted in children with cerebral palsy.

In Iraq there were actually three major outbreaks of alkylmercury poisoning. All involved consumption of seed grain that had been treated with either ethylmercury or methylmercury. The first outbreak occurred in 1956 and involved approximately 100 reported cases of poisoning. The second was more severe and took place in 1960. During the 1960 outbreak there were 1022 cases reported. The 1972 outbreak of methylmercury poisoning in Iraq involved over 6350 hospital admissions and certainly ranks as the worst catastrophe in the world involving toxic exposure to mercury in any form. There were 459 people who died in the hospital and whose deaths were directly attributed to their exposure to methylmercury. The predominant cause of poisoning was attributed to eating bread prepared from seed wheat that had been treated with a methylmercury fungicide. All of the classic symptoms and signs of methylmercury poisoning were present in both the adult and pediatric population who had eaten the poisoned bread.

The initial involvement of the Central Nervous System (CNS) in mercury intoxication usually produces the following symptoms: numbness and tingling of fingers, toes, nose and lips; fine tremor of the hands and usually the loss of ability to perform fine movements of the hand; there may also be a problem with walking, associated with ataxia. Ataxia is a condition involving the muscles that results in irregularity of muscular action or a failure of muscular coordination. There may also be a constriction or narrowing of the visual fields, and a loss of hearing. It was these initial symptoms that assisted in identifying mercury as the toxic agent involved. There was also an incident in the United States in 1969. In New Mexico a family of nine, including a pregnant woman, were poisoned by eating pork from animals that had been fed seed grain coated with methylmercury. This incident involved the fetus of the pregnant woman which is the only published report of fetal toxicity due to methylmercury poisoning occurring in the United States.

During 1983 there were eight different outbreaks of Kawaski disease reported in the United States. The disease is named after its discoverer Dr. Tomisaku Kawasaki, a Japanese pediatrician. During the Minamata and Niigata incidents there were about 50 cases of mucocutaneous lymph node syndrome (MLNS) that came to the attention of Dr. Kawasaki. All of these children presented with the same type of symptoms: fever of more than 5 days duration, conjunctivitis, pharyngitis (sore throat) with strawberry tongue, peripheral erythema (flushed skin) with subsequent desquamation truncal exanthem (eruptive fever and shedding of body skin) and cervical adenopathy (enlargement of lymph glands in the neck). Dr. Kawasaki published a report on his findings with the 50 cases and related it to mercury toxicity resulting from eating fish, although he was unable to confirm the presence of mercury in his patients. After publication of Dr. Kawasaki's report many other Japanese physicians realized that they had been encountering the same syndrome in many of their patients. A special MLNS study group was established under the auspices of the Japanese Ministry of Health and Welfare and between 1960 and 1976, nearly 10,000 cases were identified in Japan.

In 1974, The Pediatrics Journal published a report on MLNS by Dr. Kawasaki and his colleagues. As a result, physicians in this country became aware that the MLNS or Kawasaki disease had existed in this country since 1971. Since then more than 400 cases of MLNS occurring in the United States have been reported to the Center for Disease Control.

In one sense, we could say that there is no difference whether we talk about mercury in medicine or mercury in dentistry, both sciences use the metal therapeutically. However our problem is one of attempting to address mercury's use in dentistry rather than its role in environmental pollution or medicine. To this end, many of the facets of mercury toxicity as they relate to medicine will be addressed in the context of amalgam's relationship or possible relationship to signs and symptomatology that have been identified or established by the medical profession for specific disease states or conditions.

REFERENCES

1. Maurissen, J.P.J., History of mercury and mercurialism. New York State Journal of Medicine, Vol. 81, pages 1902–1909, 1981.

2. Almkvist, J., Some notes on the history of mercury intoxication. Acta Medica Scandinavica, Vol. 70, page 463, 1929.

3. Goldwater, L. J., From Hippocrates to Ramazzini: early history of industrial medicine. Annual Medical History, Vol. 8, page 27, 1936.

4. Francis, J. W., Observations on the natural and medical history of mercury. American Medical Recorder, Vol. 5, page 395, 1822.

5. Centers for Disease Control, Kawasaki disease. The Morbidity and Mortality Weekly Report, Vol. 29, pages 61–63, 1980, and Vol. 32, issue 7, pages 875–906, 1982–1983.

6. Bakir, F., et al. Methylmercury poisoning in Iraq. Science, Vol. 181, pages 230–241, 1973.

7. Elhassani, S. B. The many faces of methymercury poisoning. Journal of Toxicology Clinical Toxicology, Vol. 19, Issue 8, pages 98–100, 1983.

8. Goldwater, L. J. Mercury: A history of quicksilver. York Press, 1972, Baltimore, Maryland.

II.
THE HISTORY OF MERCURY IN DENTISTRY

The type of material utilized to fill teeth has always presented problems of one kind or another to the dental profession.

The ability to use any type of metal always presented difficulty to the dentist in the manipulation of it to "fill" a small area in a tooth. Over the years it was a constant challenge to the ingenuity and inventiveness of the dental practitioners to eliminate the difficulties of working with single metals to make them more pliable and capable of being molded (plastic) and which would then harden and have some permanence.

The first plastic metallic fillings, which had some quality of permanence, were called "fusible metals". D'Arcet's "mineral cement" was first in the field and was 8 parts bismuth, 5 parts lead, 3 parts tin, and 1/10th part of mercury to hasten the fusing process. This was used in France and first made its appearance in the United States about 1820. The problem with this material was that it had to be melted and then poured into the cavity.

It was about 1826 that M. Taveau of Paris was advocating the use of a "Silver Paste" for permanent fillings. The silver paste proposed by M. Taveau was a simple combination of silver and mercury. For convenience sake, silver coins were subsequently used instead of the purified silver. The coins were filed down and sufficient mercury added to the filings to make a paste or plastic mass. The free mercury was then pressed out and the residue was placed in the cavity where it soon hardened.

So with the refinement of M. Taveau's silver paste by using silver coin filings which also contained other metals (like copper) used in the manufacture of the coins, silver amalgam was born and ushered into the world.

However, this new silver paste exhibited some very undesirable properties when passing from a plastic state into the rigid or hardened state. The mixture would expand after setting and it was not unusual for the patient to return with a fractured tooth or the filling protruding above the cavity, which of course would be interfering with closing of the jaw. As a result, most dentists went back to using gold foil or other substances which, although they did not have the plastic quality of amalgam, were much more preferable to the dentist than coping with the problems presented by use of the silver paste.

The ability of amalgam to be manipulated was its greatest asset and ultimately scientific experimentation would have produced an amalgam without the undesireable properties of the original formulations. I say "would have" because an incident occurred in New York City that precluded this happening for almost 60 years and, in effect, started what is commonly referred to as the 1st Amalgam War.

In 1833, two brothers by the name of Crawcour suddenly appeared in New York City and began a dental practice. They were two adventurers, who had no training, experience, or skill and who exploited the use of amalgam by an unprecedented advertising campaign. The thrust of their advertising was that they had available a new material that was much cheaper than gold and did not require the same degree of painful preparation that the use of gold did.

The professional dentists rebelled for two major reasons: 1. the exploitation and use of a filling material that was totally unsatisfactory and 2. a duty to protect the public from "charlatans". Although they were quacks, without any professional credentials, the Crawcours were fierce and ruthless competitors and soon built a thriving dental practice. In fact, they were so successful, their office was filled with the best patients of the area's foremost dentists.

This would never do, of course, so the dental profession started a relentless crusade against the foreign charlatans. Amalgam was denounced not only as a poor filling material but also as the cause of mercurial poisoning, diseases of the gums and numerous other disastrous ills. The crusade was so powerful that the Crawcours were finally compelled to retire in defeat.

The amalgam war raged within the dental profession for almost 25 additional years. Organized dentistry disowned and denounced the use of amalgam. In the forefront of the war was the American Society of Dental Surgeons founded by Dr. C. A. Harris in 1840, at about the same time he opened the first dental college in the United States, The Baltimore College of Dental Surgery.

One of the first resolutions passed by the American Society

of Dental Surgeons was to the effect that "the use of lithodeen mineral paste and all other substances of which mercury is an ingredient were hurtful both to the teeth and all parts of the mouth and that there was no tooth in which caries in it could be arrested and the organ rendered serviceable by being filled, in which gold could not be employed". Members were obliged to sign pledges promising not to use amalgam upon threat of expulsion from the Society.

Some members were actually expelled from the Society because they used amalgam. In spite of this, there was a sizeable minority, particularly those dentists working for the poorer people, who paid very little attention to the resolution. Their patients could not afford gold foil fillings, and although amalgam was an unsatisfactory filling material, it was better than anything else they could use for the fees they were able to collect.

Added to all the acrimony and bitterness was a basic resentment on the part of many of the prominent dentists of admitting that a dental society had the power to make them sign pledges or suspend them for failing to sign. In 1855, in order to put an end to the internal conflicts within the Society, most of the resolutions prohibiting use of amalgam were withdrawn. The controversy over amalgam and having its membership comply finally broke up the American Society of Dental Surgeons.

About the same time, Dr. Elisha Townsend of Philadelphia proposed an amalgam consisting of 4 parts silver and 5 parts tin which were melted together. This was then reduced to filings and mixed with mercury to make a plastic mass for use in filling cavities. Other dentists also began to experiment and develop new formulas for amalgam that hopefully would overcome the expansion problems.

Under the leadership of Dr. J. Foster Flagg, the first organized movement on behalf of amalgam was begun in the late 1870's. The movement was notable for its creed that amalgam was a valuable filling material and reports of it being injurious to the health of the patient were unfounded and untrue. Most of the experiments done to prove this new creed were inconclusive and the dental profession remained in doubt as to the advisability of using amalgam for filling teeth.

This was all changed by the efforts of one man, Dr. G. V.

Black. He spent most of his years as a teacher, lecturer, and scientific researcher. Dr. Black probably contributed more to the progress of dentistry than any other single individual. The most notable of Dr. Black's achievements was the perfection of dental amalgam in the early 1900's.

The 2nd Amalgam War started shortly thereafter and is attributed almost exclusively to the efforts of one Professor Alfred Stock of Germany. Dr. Stock taught chemistry at the Kaiser-Wilheim Institute of Chemistry, and in 1926 he elected to publish his own personal experiences with mercury, which had destroyed a major part of his life. Dr. Stock's exposure to mercury was in the laboratory in the course of teaching and chemical experimentation over 25 years.

From our standpoint, what was most significant about Dr. Stock's 1926 article, was the identification of silver amalgam fillings in the mouth as a source of mercury vapor. Moreover, he outlined the scientific experiments that confirmed his findings. Dr. Stock concluded his article with the following paragraph "Dentistry should completely avoid the use of amalgam for fillings or at least not use it whenever this is possible. There is no doubt that many symptoms: tiredness, depression, irritability, vertigo, weak memory, mouth inflamations, diarrhea, loss of appetite and chronic catarrhs often are caused by mercury which the body is exposed to from amalgam fillings, in small amounts, but continuously. Doctors should give this fact their serious consideration. It will then likely be found that the thoughtless introduction of amalgam as a filling material for teeth was a severe sin against humanity".

With that article started the second amalgam war. Charges and counter charges were the order of the day and this continued on (in fact it's still going on) until events of World War II temporarily halted the arguments. Stock continued his research, and in 1939 published an article outlining further facts about amalgam. He identified it as an unstable alloy that continuously gave off mercury in the form of gas ions and abraded particles. Stock's articles created consternation among the metallurgists, doctors, dentists, and chemists and were reported in great detail in the press. Dr. Frykholm states that at a lecture in Sweden in 1941, Stock modified his position by claiming that the rare cases of mercury poisoning caused by mercury vapor leaching out of amalgam restorations should not affect the further use of silver amalgam in dental practice. This appears to be an error or misinterpretation made by Dr. Frykholm in the translation of that speech. In another translation made by Mats Hanson and stated in a presentation he made at a seminar on mercury toxicity given in Colorado in September of 1983, Hanson stated that Stock reaffirmed his position that amalgam was highly toxic and should not be used by the dental profession as a restoration material.

Whose translation is correct is immaterial because all of Stock's research findings related to amalgam and mercury have essentially been confirmed. The latest in 1984.

After World War II, the world went about the business of picking up the pieces and getting on with life. However, it wasn't long before the continued use of mercury in dentistry evoked those same passionate pro or con amalgam positions within the dental and scientific communities. Behind it all of course was Stock's work and the burning questions raised by him: Does mercury actually escape from dental amalgam fillings? If it does escape, does it do any damage to the human body?

Enter the "3rd Amalgam War". A war that is still in progress and will continue on until organized dentistry, medicine, and "the establishment" either accept the anti-amalgam position with its overwhelming array of documented scientific research or, once and for all times, provide incontrovertible proof that mercury in amalgam does not escape from the filling material once it is in the tooth or, that if any mercury does escape that it is not toxic to the human body in continuous micro dosages.

The battle was joined, on many fronts and in many countries of the world. In order for you to have a better grasp of some of the battles and on what battlefields they were and are being fought the following overview is provided.

The American Dental Association which came into being at about the same time the American Society of Dental Surgeons was being dissolved, supported the use of silver amalgam then as the restoration material of choice and still does today. I suppose Psychiatrists or Psychologists might be able to explain why certain officials of this fine professional association adhere so vehemently to a policy that continues to champion the use of mercury amalgam. Or they might advance some acceptable rationale that would also explain why these same individuals go out of their way to denigrate the use of non-toxic replacement materials for posterior restorations, when such materials are available today and in fact, are comparable or superior to amalgam.

I wholeheartedly champion the doctrine of reasonable doubt. The scientific community should take a lesson from the courts of law in this regard and if there is a reasonable doubt that a substance may be injurious to the human organism, its use should be stopped. It just doesn't make sense to continue the use of a product that is known to be one of the most toxic to man when there are suitable substitutes that at this point in time can be considered non-toxic.

In regard to the use of composite materials for posterior restorations there seems to be a double standard being applied by the ADA in accepting materials for inclusion in their list of approved filling materials. The new composites are being subjected to very rigid standards requiring up to seven years of testing in the mouth in addition to meeting the basic structural requirements. Conversely, it appears that new amalgam formulations are being approved if they meet the structural requirements, as over 100 different amalgams are on their approved list. If each required 7 years of testing I don't think any of them could survive the wait.

This lack of acceptance of the newer composites by the ADA has some serious overtones. Insurance companies are using this fact to deny payment of claims where the dentist has used the new composites for posterior restorations. This is truly an unfortunate situation which only hurts the patient. The new composites show greater structural strength than amalgam and have exhibited wear characteristics that are close to that of amalgam.

I was always under the impression that it was the dentist who went to college to learn his profession and that once he had graduated and had been licensed to practice dentistry in his particular state, it was the dentist's decision how best to treat his patient. I must be wrong because we now have the situation where the insurance companies and the ADA determine what the dentist can do. It is not price that the insurance companies are objecting to but rather that the composite materials being used for posterior restorations are not on the ADA list of approved materials.

The ADA also appears to have some problem in accepting the findings of some research papers. Articles published in non-United States scientific journals do not seem to command the same attention and acceptance than those articles published in U.S. Journals do. That is with the exception of those articles that support the ADA position on mercury amalgam.

It is extremely interesting that any scientific article refuting Stock's work seems to be acceptable to the ADA while the great volume of scientific evidence confirming Stock's work is ignored or the implications are that the research was flawed.

This is especially true when you consider that the major work of Dr. Karl O. Frykholm, published in Acta Odontologica Scandinavica in Stockholm Sweden in 1957, has been the cornerstone of the American Dental Association's policy that amalgam is safe except in those few individuals who may be hypersensitive to mercury. All of the published articles based on experiments that utilized much more sophisticated equipment than that used by Dr. Frykholm and which arrived at conclusions contrary to Frykholm's have been totally ignored by the ADA, or interpreted in such a manner that the conclusions supported the ADA position.

REFERENCES

1. History of dental and oral science in America, prepared under direction of the American Academy of Dental Science, Published by Samuel S. White, 1876, Philadelphia, Pennsylvania.

2. Bremmer, D. K., The Story of Dentistry, revised 3rd edition, 1954. Dental Items of Interest Publishing Co., Inc., Brooklyn, N.Y.

3. Stock, A., The Hazards of Mercury Vapor. Zeitsch Angew Chem, Vol. 39, pages 461–488, 1926.

4. Hanson, M., Nothing New Under The Sun: Experiences with Mercury Poisoning Related by Dr. Alfred Stock and Dr. E. Jaensch in 1926. Journal of Orthomolecular Psychiatry, Vol. 12, issue 3, pages 355–358, 1983.

5. Frykholm, K. O., On Mercury from Dental Amalgam: Its Toxic and Allergic Effects and some Comments on Occupational Hygiene. Acta Odontologica Scandanivica, Vol. 22, Supplement 22, pages 1–123, 1957.

6. Flagg, J. F., The Choice of Proper Filling Material, 1900.

CHAPTER 2

WHERE ARE WE NOW?

You should be made aware of the magnitude of the problems related to research and the dissemination of research findings. The type of research we are speaking of involves those areas that have the potential to impact on man as a species and to affect his survival.

The complexity of the problem is mind boggling. To place it in some sort of perspective, let's look at the problem of heart disease and take the thousands of papers that have been published on this particular subject as an example:

Problem 1. These papers have been published in hundreds of different journals and books all over the world.

Problem 2. There is no universal language for the publication of scientific research. Consequently, if a Russian scientist should publish his findings on an aspect of heart disease that has taken years of scientific experimentation, it would be written in Russian and published in a Russian journal or book. It might languish there for years until some other government, company, or individual discovers it and ascertains it is worthy of translation into their language. Here in the United States, a great percentage of this translation is done under sponsorship of the concerned agency of the federal government. It is then published by the U.S. Government Printing Office and made available to the public at a price. How does Dr. Jones the cardiologist practicing in Los Angeles, know that the government has just published a major Russian research work on heart disease? The only way he would ever find out is if one of the American journals he subscribes to happened to have a researcher and/or reporter who became aware of the translated Russian paper and thought it was significant enough to do an article about it.

Problem 3. The average health professional usually subscribes to all of the publications related to his specialty or particular area of interest. Finding time to read them is another matter. Some have their staff skim the articles and point out the ones that they should read. Others just pile them up in stacks, promising themselves they will take time to go through them. His time is taken up not only in attending to his patients, but he is actually running a business and must devote a percentage of his time to business matters. Then there is his family and social obligations and the requirement to attend seminars or formal classes that are a part of his profession's continuing education requirement to maintain professional standing. Last, but not least, there is always the spector of a malpractice suit hanging over his head and additional time must be spent in insuring everything that could have been done, has in fact been done.

Problem 4. If an individual had nothing to do except read 12 hours a day, it would probably take him six months to find and read everything that was published TODAY that pertained to his specialty or area of interest. By the time he finished reading the information published today, it would have been updated or superseded by hundreds of other articles.

Problem 5. The answer to a problem may be obscured. There are literally thousands of enzyme systems in the body. A team of 5 medical doctors and biochemists have just spent 2 years researching one enzyme system. They have documented everything it does and how it does it and its interrelationships to various other functions and organs, glands, blood, muscles, etc. etc.. They have also determined which amino acids, vitamins, minerals, hormones, etc., are affected by this enzyme. Truly a remarkable and historical research effort. However, unknown to them, another team of researchers is investigating the impact of various drugs (normally prescribed) on this same particular enzyme system. Their results indicate that if you take Drug A, it will inhibit the enzyme from performing its normal functions. What they didn't know was that still another group, testing the same drug, reached a conclusion that it had no effect at all on that particular enzyme system. Confused? Wait! The three reports are published individually in three different journals, only one of which your doctor subscribes to. Wait!!! There is more. As soon as the article is published, doctors and scientists all over the world who are familiar with the subject and/or have been doing their own independent research, write in and either point out what they consider to be flaws in the basic protocol used for the research, or tell of their own experiences using the drug, which are contrary to the information published. If your doctor had only read one of the articles, how could he make an informed judgment? That analogy would apply to a great many of today's dentists who continue to use mercury amalgam fillings. They have just not been exposed to the preponderance of scientific data that would permit them to make a rational personal judgement on the subject.

Problem 6. Don't bother me with the facts! The high ego, authoritarian health professional will sometimes find published articles so contrary to his training and beliefs that he totally closes his mind to the fact that they might be true. Can you blame him? What would you do if you had spent from 5 to 14 years studying a particular way of doing something and you were even recognized as an expert in your field, and suddenly you are confronted with evidence done in a laboratory with test tubes and animals that implies everything you have been doing and advocating is wrong? I am sure you would resist or even try to set up research projects to prove you weren't wrong, or to find evidence refuting the findings contrary to your own. How can you blame the physician, who received 3 hours of instruction on nutrition out of 8 years of formal training, for laughing when you ask him whether nutrition would help cure your particular problem. By the same token, how can you blame your dentist for putting silver amalgam in your mouth when it has been used for over 150 years for that very purpose? In both instances it is only in recent years that researchers have had available to them large computerized data bases that have permitted the review and correlation of data from multiple disciplines. Even with the data available, it is an awesome task correlating information from biochemistry, chemistry, metallurgy, electrochemistry, pathology, physiology, neurology, pharmacology, toxicology, etc., and then interpreting and assembling the results of your research into cohesive statements. For example, the information upon which this book is being written, is based on research articles compiled over a 2½ year span.

Problem 7. How do you ascertain if something proven in a laboratory with sophisticated analytical machinery, test tubes, chemicals, and animals is true in the human body? Fortunately, you can't go around killing human beings and dissecting and assaying their bodies. Therefore, some things can never be proven to the satisfaction of the pure scientist. As a rule, the scientific world does not accept anecdotal evidence as proof. What this means is that if you had a serious health problem and took a particular vitamin, or performed a certain type of exercise, or only ate certain foods and you got better, that would be an anecdote and not a scientific fact. To be scientific you would have to have a double blind study. This is where two groups of patients are established, all with similar symptoms and all within the same age grouping. One group is given placebos (sugar pills) and the other is given the actual vitamin. Neither group nor the investigators knows what they are taking. At the end of the test period, the results are analyzed and a conclusion is drawn from the results as to the efficacy of the vitamin.

Why have I belabored the problems related to research? The answer is quite simple—our current situation with silver amalgam. There is a substantial flow of anecdotal evidence being reported by dentists and physicians who believe that the research to date has indicated with sufficient clarity that amalgams in teeth may be injurious to our health. These health practitioners have recommended removal of amalgam fillings and replacement with new composite materials (composed of quartz or other fillers and certain plastic compounds) that are basically non-toxic. Where the patient has agreed to this type of reconstruction and the work was performed, there has usually been an abatement, amelioration or complete clearing of symptoms. This is not true in all cases because here again we are dealing with the most complex piece of machinery in the world, "The Human Body", and we are all different biochemically. Questions such as: How long has the problem existed? Has irreparable damage been done which cannot be corrected by removing or correcting the cause of the problem? Is there another cause existant at the same time? And on and on.

On the other side of the problem we have the proponents who advocate continued use of amalgam fillings. The combined credentials and strength of this group is awesome. It includes the National Institute of Dental Research, National Bureau of Standards, The American Dental Association (ADA), The Academy of General Dentistry (AGD), most of the state dental societies, all of the teaching college and university dental schools and most of the medical doctors. Although the ADA in reality is only a professional association, they in effect set the acceptable standards for the dental industry.

Of the 100,000 plus practicing dentists in the United States, there is only a small minority at this time (somewhere in the order of 2000) who do not accept the ADA position on the use of amalgam in dentistry. The official ADA position on this problem as expressed in the Journal of the American Dental Association, Vol 106, April, 1983, is summarized in the following quote: "The Association wishes to emphasize that except in individuals sensitive to mercury, there is no reason why a patient should seek at this time to have amalgam restorations (silver fillings) removed. Indeed, the effect of such a procedure and further restorative operations could be detrimental to the patients oral health, including the unnecessary loss of teeth and cannot be justified." There are several things about that statement that bother me, not the least of which is the question of for whom the article was being written? Doesn't it seem kind of strange that in a professional journal for dentists, the "unnamed authors" would have to parenthetically explain to the doctors that amalgam restorations meant "silver fillings"???

The last point aside, you can see that we do have a real conflict and difference of opinion. Each side is armed with published scientific research, in many instances the same research, that is being interpreted as supporting their position.

WHAT TO DO?

The balance of this book will try to tell the story of the research that has been published. We will try to relate, in terms and language that a non-technical person can understand, both sides of the debate and let you be the final judge. Your decision may be influenced to some degree by your own health status and whether anyone up till now has been able to give you a satisfactory answer as to what is causing your condition or problem, if you have a health condition or problem.

CHAPTER 3

WHAT IS MERCURY?

At this point, it is extremely important to attempt to define what mercury or quicksilver (as it is sometimes called) really is.

Mercury is a highly toxic silver-white, liquid metal which is highly volatile at ordinary temperatures and the fumes of which are readily absorbed when inhaled.

Is all mercury toxic or injurious to our health? The answer is an unqualified yes. Some forms of this metal are much more toxic than others. In this book we will deal with the two main groupings of mercury compounds, inorganic and organic.

INORGANIC MERCURY

Within this group there is: elemental mercury, elemental mercury vapor, elemental mercurous and mercuric salts and some complexes of the mercuric ions that can form reversible bonds with certain tissue ligands such as thiol groups on protein. The last statement merely means that once inside your body, the mercury can attach itself to sulfur containing compounds that are part of a protein molecule. In other words it is a hitchhiker who has caught a ride on a vehicle that is part of a pretty sophisticated transport system that travels to all parts of our bodies.

We can absorb inorganic mercury by inhalation of the vapor from elemental mercury or aerosols of mercuric salts. It can enter orally or be absorbed through the skin, mucous membranes and digestive tract.

Elemental mercury is the most volatile form of the metal because it readily gives off vapor when agitated, compressed, heated, or exposed to the air at normal temperature. Elemental mercury is used in dentistry to make the silver amalgam fillings. It is also found in barometers, thermometers and medical instruments. Our concern with elemental mercury relates to any exposure to the vapors given off, because the vapor is so readily absorbed by our bodies when inhaled. Diffusion of elemental mercury vapor into the tissues and across cell membranes is facilitated by its lipid solubility (will mix with fats) and its lack of an electrical charge. The electrical charge, whether positive or negative, has a lot to do with how different materials get in and out of our cells to do the jobs nature designed for them.

Mercurous Chloride is the best known of the mercurous compounds. It is sometimes referred to as Calomel which for years was used as a cathartic but is not used anymore. It is, however, still used in some skin creams as an antiseptic. Mercurous Iodide was once used as a treatment for syphilis.

Mercuric salts are a very irritating and toxic form of the metal. Mercuric chloride is used as an antiseptic and is very toxic when swallowed. In fact, it is so toxic that it was one of the preferred poisons with which to commit suicide with. Mercurochrome and thiomersal (merthiolate) utilized as antiseptics are considered by the medical profession to be relatively safe because of the dilute solution and the fact that the solution is less soluble and doesn't penetrate the skin easily. Once again, current information is drastically changing this opinion. The FDA has recently published an advisory concerning the death of a child who was being treated with merthiolate for an infection in her ear. As a result, the FDA is now proposing regulatory change that would forbid the use of mercury in any over-the-counter product.

Mercuric salts are still widely employed in industry today. Waste from these industries is discharged into nearby rivers, thus polluting them in many parts of the world.

Continued exposure to mercuric salts can cause neurological and behavioral changes. The phrase "He is Mad as a

Hatter'' and the character of the Mad Hatter in Lewis Carrol's Alice's Adventures in Wonderland, stem from the "changes" that used to happen to people who worked in the felt hat industry. If you recall, in the chapter on medical history, we said that an important event occurred towards the end of the 17th century. In 1685, mercury nitrate began to be used in France in the preparation of fur felt. The mercury nitrate was used in the carrotting process in making fur felt for the hats.

ORGANIC MERCURY

This group of compounds are also called organomercurials and as with the inorganic mercury, toxicity varies depending upon the particular compound. Within this grouping alkylmercurials are considered the most dangerous. They can enter the body by inhalation, skin absorption or oral ingestion. They are volatile and exposure to their vapors can readily occur. They are also lipid soluble (this means they will dissolve in fats normally available in our bodies) and readily cross biological membranes making for highly toxic potentials.

Alkylmercury salts have been widely used as fungicides. Use as such has led to major incidents of human poisoning from the inadvertent consumption of mercury treated seed grain. The worst incident occurred in Iraq in 1972. Wheat and barley seed grain that had been treated with methylmercury was distributed for use in planting only. Instead, the grain was ground into flour and made into bread. As a result, approximately 6500 people were hospitalized and 500 died.

Methylmercury is very volatile. So much so that it is chemically reduced to be used as a liquid or solid aerosol spray. When inhaled in the form of aerosols, these compounds are likely to dissolve quickly in body fluids and be distributed to the blood.

Phenyl mercuric propionate is used as an antimildew additive. It is incorporated in many of the water based paints used on exteriors. It is a potentially dangerous source of mercury intoxication that could result from inhalation of its toxic vapors.

To give you some idea of the overall mercury pollution problem, let's look at the following facts:

CHLORINE AND ALKALI PRODUCERS. For every ton of chlorine produced, nearly half a pound of mercury escapes into the environment. This adds up to about 1,200,000 pounds a year.

AGRICULTURE. About 1,000,000 pounds a year are used as fungicides protecting our seed grains and as insecticides spraying our plants.

COAL BURNING. The average mercury content of coal is about 0.3 parts per million. Of this, approximately 95% is expelled in flue gases during combustion. World atmospheric contamination by coal burning is estimated to be about 6–10 million lbs. per year.

VOLCANOES. Mercury also enters the world oceans from this source.

Overall, it is estimated that 20,000,000 pounds of mercury flow into the sea each year, half of this of natural origin and the other half from industrial sources. It would take years to document all of the industrial users of mercury around the world and calculate their contributions to the overall pollution problem. I think it would be safe to assume that the foregoing information represents only the tip of the iceberg.

So far, we have provided little information relating to the main purpose of writing this book. It is not a crusade against mercury per se but is intended to forcefully bring out the point that our total body burden of mercury can come from many sources. The fact has a very specific relationship to be considered by you when making your final judgement about the dental and medical professions use of mercury.

Do dentists use a a lot of mercury? Present estimates are that approximately 250,000 lbs. a year are being used in the U.S. alone and that by the year 2000, this figure could be 600,000 lbs. That's a lot of mercury going into the mouths/bodies of human beings.

As we have stated previously, our major health concern really centers around inhaling vapours from elemental mercury and methylmercury vapor from organic mercury. The heart of the controversy swirling around the use of silver amalgam as a dental filling material, is the essential and critical answer which you as an individual with mercury amalgam fillings in your mouth must reach is: "Has my personal health or the health of my family been adversely affected because of these controversial fillings?'' So that YOU and not some un-named committee of an association can make this important decision, the following chapter will attempt to provide you with all the arguments being used FOR and AGAINST the continued use of mercury amalgam as the desired dental filling material.

REFERENCES

1. Arena, J. M., Poisoning, 4th edition, 1979, Charles C. Thomas, Springfield, Illinois, 1979.

2. Goodman and Gillman's, The Pharmacological Basis of Therapeutics, 6th edition, 1980, The Macmillan Publishing Co., Inc., New York.

3. Safety of Dental Amalgam, Journal American Dental Association, 106:74–76, 1983.

4. Seese, W. S., and Daub, G. H., Basic Chemistry, 2nd Edition, 1977, Prentice-Hall, Inc., Englewood Cliffs, N.J.

5. Dickey, L. D. (Ed), Clinical Ecology, Charles C. Thomas, Springfield, Illinois, 1976.

6. Billings, C. E., and Matson, W. R., Mercury Emissions from Coal Combustion, Science, 176:1232, 1972.

7. Schroeder, H. S., The Poisons Around Us, Keats Publishing, New Canaan, CT., 1974.

8. Land Yearbook, U.S. Department of Agriculture, 1958.

9. Minerals Yearbook, U.S. Bureau of Mines, 1972.

10. A Recommended Standard for Occupational Exposure to Inorganic Mercury, USDHEW, Public Health Service, National Institute for Occupational Safety and Health (NIOSH), 1973.

CHAPTER 4

THE ARGUMENTS FOR AND AGAINST

The FOR position as expressed in each one of the following arguments represents a position of the American Dental Association and/or the proponents of continued use of amalgam that are referenced by the ADA, and/or those research papers that the ADA has interpreted to be supportive of their position. Where available I have cited the scientific references used as a basis for the ADA position taken.

I should point out at this time an idiosyncrasy of the ADA that disturbs me. The No-Author/No-Name position/policy papers published by the ADA. Most of the important decisions and policies published by the ADA in their Journal or Newspaper show the author as the "Council on Dental Materials, Instruments and Equipment; Council on Dental Therapeutics; or Bureau of Economic Research and Statistics". I should think that of the more than 100,000 dentists who are members of the ADA, someone would complain and insist that the names of the Council or Bureau members (certainly the Chairman or Head) be printed in the article or in each issue. Certainly the dentists, or at the very least we the patients, are entitled to know who (and even possibly what their qualifications are) is making all of these decisions for an entire profession that can have such a bearing on the health of an entire population.

It is paradoxical that the dentists of 1850 rebelled against their Association, The American Society of Dental Surgeons, because the Society was attempting to dictate to them what filling material they could use. Here we are in 1984, and nobody seems to be questioning the right of the American Dental Association to dictate to them; not even those whose voices are raised in protest against the continued use of amalgam. Their fight is against the use of amalgam and not the right of a professional association to dictate policy.

Immediately following the FOR positions, I have listed the AGAINST positions. These are the answers derived only from published scientific research papers, articles, or books, that can be considered as reflecting conclusions contrary to those taken by the American Dental Association. The information contained in the AGAINST positions essentially represents the facts being used by those dentists who have made their individual decisions to stop using mercury amalgam in their dental practice.

You, the reader, must be the final judge of which position is right or wrong because, in the end, it is you who should make the important decision: "YES," please put some more poison in my body because I agree with you that there really isn't a reasonable doubt that it can harm me in any way. Or "NO," there is enough evidence it can harm me. The burden of proof is on you and not me. You must prove to my satisfaction that it is safe to put in my body. The doctrine of reasonable doubt must prevail. If you cannot prove beyond a reasonable doubt that the mercury you want to put in my mouth will not be damaging to my body now or at some future date, then I must insist that you do not place more amalgam fillings in my mouth. I would also like you to remove and replace my existing mercury amalgam fillings with something other than a known poison. I understand that you cannot provide me with unequivocal scientific proof that mercury is not harming my body. However, because it is my body, I am willing to accept "anecdotal" evidence as proof of reasonable doubt!

ARGUMENT 1
THE AMERICAN DENTAL ASSOCIATION IS
CONSTANTLY STUDYING AND EVALUATING THE
SAFETY AND TOLERANCE OF MERCURY USED IN
DENTAL RESTORATIONS

SOURCE: Journal of the American Dental Association
(JADA), Vol 106, April 1983.

TITLE: Safety of Dental Amalgam

AUTHOR: Council on Dental Materials, Instruments and
Equipment
Council on Dental Therapeutics

STATEMENT: "The Councils have received several inquiries regarding the continued use of dental amalgam and the practice by some of removing amalgam restorations and replacing them with gold alloy castings or composite restorative materials. Dental amalgam is used in approximately 75% of the single tooth restorations. The use of mercury in these restorations is constantly being studied and evaluated for its safety and tolerance."

FOR: The last sentence in the statement puts forth a policy position that the ADA is constantly studying the use of mercury in restorations for safety and tolerance. Unfortunately, the ADA cites no references to indicate research that the association has done and/or sponsored to support the policy position. As a result I can only conclude that the Council assumes their normal conduct of business reflects that position.

AGAINST: I was unable to find any published research finding of primary research that had been done by the ADA. However further along in the source article, the ADA states that they have two existing programs to investigate the effects of high levels of mercury vapor on the health of dental personnel. These programs are not designed to investigate the potential toxic effects of dental amalgam fillings. They are only designed to measure the amount of mercury in the urine of participating dentists associated with their exposure to mercury in their normal work environment. As for safety and tolerance in the patient, they cite (elsewhere in the source article) an article published in the June 1982 issue of the California Dental Association Journal, which consisted of a review of existing literature. This particular article presents evidence which appears to be contrary to the authors' conclusions which stated that the use of amalgams in fillings is relatively safe.

I am unable to judge what is the exact meaning of the term "relatively safe," in its application to the health of hundreds of millions of people.

ARGUMENT 2
DENTISTRY NEED ONLY CONCERN ITSELF WITH THE POTENTIAL TOXICITY OF MERCURY VAPOR

SOURCE: JADA, Vol 106, April 1983.
TITLE: Safety of Dental Amalgam.
AUTHOR: Council on Dental Materials, Instruments and Equipment
Council on Dental Therapeutics
STATEMENT: "An international committee on the hazards of mercury, classified mercury and it compounds in the order of their decreasing toxicity: first, methyl and ethyl mercury compounds, next mercury vapor, and last the inorganic salts as well as a number of organic forms. The toxic potential of these forms of mercury in dentistry is limited to mercury vapor."
FOR: Here again, the ADA does not cite any references to support the last sentence which is their policy position. I would have to assume that they are basing their statement on the work of Dr. K. O. Frykholm published in 1957. Dr. Frykholm concluded from his experiments that a small transient amount of mercury vapor escapes from newly installed amalgam fillings but that it only lasts for about a week and is not a problem. Which would then leave the main focus of the ADA's concern to be the mercury vapor that may be present in the dental office environment. There concern here centers around the fact that the elemental mercury utilized to make the amalgam is highly volatile and gives off mercury vapor when exposed to normal room temperature which is increased during the normal process of handling and mixing. In this regard, the ADA has been extremely effective in educating dental personnel as to the hazards of mercury vapor and has published many fine articles on the subject over the years.

AGAINST: The classification of the different forms of mercury in their order of toxicity is correct. The statement concerning dentistry's concern being only with mercury vapor is incorrect. Dentistry must be concerned with methylmercury, the most toxic of the various forms of mercury, because of biological processes that can transform the mercury vapor in the body into methyl mercury. These processes are biotransformation and methylation.

Biotransformation: Elemental mercury (this is the kind used in dentistry) produces mercury vapor. This fact has never been disputed. What has always been questioned is that mercury amalgam once installed in a tooth gives off mercury vapor. Dr. Stock demonstrated this in 1926 and published papers detailing his experiments and findings. Dr. Stock's original findings have been confirmed by several researchers the latest of which are: Dr. Gay and associates in 1979; Dr. Reinhardt and associates in 1979; and Dr. Svare and associates in 1981. These groups of researchers measured the amount of mercury vapor in the mouth before and after chewing gum for 10 minutes and have produced scientific proof that amalgams give off mercury vapor during the normal processes of chewing and swallowing.

Now we have established the fact that there is a continuous source of mercury vapor. When mercury vapor is inhaled there is a very rapid and efficient absorption of it by the lungs. Depending upon the amount being inhaled, the absorption rate can be from 74% for large amounts and up to 100% for small amounts. (Berlin, et al, 1969, Kudak, F. Nielsen 1965). Once absorbed, about 30% of the mercury vapor is transferred to the blood within 10 minutes. (Berlin, et al, 1969).

It is at this point that biotransformation begins. Some of the mercury vapor remains unchanged and some of it is oxidized. (This means to remove a pair of hydrogen atoms and to combine with oxygen. Chemically it means the increase of a positive electrical charge and the decrease of the negative charge which in effect ionizes the vapor). The unchanged portion exists dissolved in the blood lipids (fats). The toxic effects are produced by that portion that is oxidized into mercuric ions which occurs partly in the blood, partly in the tissues but mainly in the erythrocytes (which most of us know by the more common name of red blood cells or corpuscles). (Clarkson, 1972).

Where does methylation come in? This presents a much more technical set of circumstances and involves organisms and bacteria found in the mouth and in the gut. It all begins with the amalgam filling in the mouth. Once installed in your tooth, there are several different factors that impact on the longevity of the filling: chewing, which exerts a tremendous compaction pressure and also tends to generate heat; saliva, which represents the acid level of your oral fluids which are also considered as electrolytes—the dissimilar metals contained in the amalgam are capable of generating electrical current between themselves and/or between adjacent filled teeth or teeth with crowns made of gold or other metal; then there are the problems associated with the acids contained in many of the foods we like to eat and drink, especially coffee, tea, and colas and the increased heat from hot liquids, foods and smoking, causing an increase in the vaporization. The filling, made of an unstable alloy to start with, is subjected to all of these various factors and forces. It begins to corrode and, as a result, not only continually gives off mercury in the form of vapor but also as mercuric ions and abraded particles. So we now have transport of a portion of the mercury into the stomach along with the food and liquid.

Several researchers, beginning with Jernelov in 1969, have demonstrated the microbial conversion or methylation of mercury by various microorganisims. This was demonstrated in the laboratory as well as inside the bodies of animals (Abdulla, et al 1973). In 1975, the methylation of mercuric chloride in human feces was demonstrated by Edwards and McBride. It was also in 1975 that Rowland, Grasso and Davies determined that most strains of staphlylococci, streptococci, yeasts and escherichia-coli found in the human intestine (these are bacteria and yeasts of different forms and shapes that are normally present in the human gut) were capable of methylating mercury. It was in 1983 that Heintze and his associates made the startling discovery that various forms of oral streptococci common in dental plaque and saliva could also methylate mercury being released from the amalgam fillings.

Based on the above stated facts, I must conclude that the ADA policy position regarding dentistry being concerned only with mercury vapor is incorrect.

ARGUMENT 3
RECENT TEST INDICATING THE RELEASE OF MERCURY VAPOR FROM DENTAL AMALGAMS IN TEETH MAY NOT BE VALID

SOURCE: JADA, Vol 106, April 1983.
TITLE: Safety of Dental Amalgam
AUTHOR: Council on Dental Materials, Instruments and Equipment
Council on Dental Therapeutics.

STATEMENT: "The dental profession is continuously evaluating the implications of exposure to mercury vapor. This attention is stimulated by the potential "body burden" of mercury from food and other sources along with the accumulations from dental treatment. The release of mercury vapor from dental amalgam in the mouth has recently been reported. (1) This information was obtained with measuring devices that show detectable amounts of mercury vapor in expired air which was collected immediately after chewing on old as well as new amalgam restorations. The authors do not indicate that the air was exhaled through the nose or mouth. If through the mouth, there is no evidence that the measurable mercury vapor was from the lungs or just the oral cavity." (The footnoted reference [1] is the article by Dr. Svare and associates published in Sept. 1981).

FOR: The "body burden" of mercury derived from our food supply and other sources is certainly a major cause for continued concern. Although no references were cited by the ADA, there have been a great number of studies done that indicate in the normal course of eating and breathing we can contribute to our total body burden of mercury. The significance of whether measurements were made while the test patients were breathing through their nose or mouth relates to the basic fact that by breathing through the nose, no air from the lungs would be passing through the oral cavity and the measurement of any mercury vapor present would accurately reflect any vapor coming from amalgams. Conversley, if the patients were breathing through their mouth, the measurements might be contaminated by vapor being expired from the lungs.

AGAINST: The Councils appear to be making some valid points in their statement. However, and for your benefit, let's take a close look at the statement sentence by sentence and really see what they are saying. "The dental profession is continuously evaluating the implications of exposure to mercury vapor. This attention is stimulated by the potential "body burden" of mercury from food and other sources along with any accumulations from dental treatment." When the Councils use the phrase the "dental profession", I personally have a serious problem in attempting to determine who in the dental profession is being stimulated by the potential body burden from food and other sources. Although not referenced directly in the source document, the ADA appears to be indirectly (through the article published by Drs. Bauer and First) referencing the work of Dr. Stofen, published in the Toxicology Journal in 1974, to support their position. In this article, Dr. Stofen states that even though mercury may be released from amalgam restorations, the amount is equal to the amount ingested through food consumption and is therefore of little concern. The rationale behind this comparison eludes me. It could mean that if one ounce of poison doesn't appear to do any damage then certainly two ounces won't harm you either.

The last part of the second sentence also addresses accumulations from dental treatment. I don't know what the Councils mean by that statement except by implication. I do know that over the years their official position has been that the patient is only exposed while the restoration is being placed in the mouth. This position, I am assuming, is based on the findings of Dr. Frykholm who concluded that mercury vapor was only released from new fillings for 5 days. After that time the filling had hardened and sealed and did not constitute a problem. By "accumulation" they must mean only those mercury particles and mercury vapor present during the first five days. That seems to be a correct interpretation because in their next three sentences they imply that the research indicating mercury is released from old fillings is flawed and that the mercury vapor measured was probably being exhaled from the lungs of the patients being tested. What this leaves the reader with is an impression that we normally exhale mercury everytime we breathe; which in some of us may be true. (A complete analysis of Dr. Frykholm's article will be provided in subsequent arguments).

This leaves us with only the problem of examining the validity of Dr. Svare's findings, and the questioning of them by the ADA. Dr. Svare's article was published in the Journal of Dental Research, Vol 60, Sept. 1981. His co-authors Drs. Reinhardt, Petersen, Boyer, Frank, Gay and Cox, had all been involved since 1978 in testing the hypothesis that amalgam restorations release mercury vapor. To a large degree, these researchers were validating the findings of Dr. Stock published in 1926. They were confirming his findings through exact measurements utilizing advanced instrumentation designed solely for the purpose of measuring the mercury vapor content of air. More importantly, they were able to gain these measurements in experiments that parallel normal use of our teeth; i.e., chewing and not chewing.

The design of the experiment involved the taking of mercury vapor measurements, or readings, in the mouth before chewing and after chewing gum for 10 minutes. There were two groups of test patients in the experiment: the controls, or individuals without any fillings of any kind in their mouths, and the second group of patients who all had amalgam fillings in their teeth. In the control group without fillings, the researchers were able to detect very small amounts of mercury vapor before chewing gum. After chewing gum for 10 minutes, the amount of mercury vapor measured in the expired breath remained the same—NO CHANGE. In the test group with amalgam fillings in their teeth, measureable amounts of mercury vapor were detected before they began chewing gum. After chewing gum for 10 minutes the researchers discovered a 15.5-fold increase in the amount of mercury vapor in their breath.

It seems that Dr. Svare and his associates demonstrated in a very clear concise way that mercury vapor is continuously being released in the mouth and that this condition is greatly aggravated by the normal processes of chewing or eating. The ADA or the Councils would have us believe by the way the policy position is phrased, that the mercury was really being exhaled out of the lungs and not being released from the amalgam filled teeth. If that were true, then the researchers should have been able to duplicate the results in the mouths of those people who had no fillings because that is what the ADA is in effect saying. Which, of course the study showed could not be done.

Even without the fact that there were no changes in the readings within the control group, the ADA offers no logical explanation as to why the group with amalgams had an increased amount of mercury vapor in their breath. Certainly they don't want us to believe that the simple act of chewing gum increases the release of mercury from our lungs. Or do they?

It is quite possible that the Councils' basic assumption put forth in the statement was founded in the fact that scientific experiments have demonstrated that a percentage of an ingested dose of mercury is exhaled in the lungs. One such experiment was conducted by Drs. Hursh, Clarkson, Cherian, Vostal and Vandermallie in 1976. In their study, they exposed 5 human volunteers to radioactive mercury vapor and concluded: the subjects retained an average of 74% of the mercury inhaled; of the 74% that was retained in the body, 7% was lost in the expired air and that the half-life of the retained mercury was 18 hours.

The term half-life is utilized to define the length of time required for living tissue or organisms to eliminate one-half of a radioactive substance which has been introduced into the body. The remaining half will have the same half-life as the original. This means that in their experiment, every 18 hours one-half of the amount remaining will be eliminated. For example, if the 74% retained amounted to 80 micrograms, after 18 hours the body would have gotten rid of 40 micrograms. Of the 40 micrograms remaining after 18 more hours had passed (total of 36 hours) 20 micrograms more would be lost leaving 20 micrograms. This goes on until all of the mercury has been dissipated.

It is possible, depending upon the amount of mercury contained in the food we eat or in the air we breathe, to have some detectable level of mercury in our expired breath. However, there is one final point I would like to make on this subject. It is extremely noble for the Councils to be concerned about our potential body burden of mercury that may be derived from food and other sources. IT HAS ABSOLUTELY NOTHING TO DO WITH DETERMINING THE SAFETY OF DENTAL AMALGAM.

ARGUMENT 4
THERE IS NO SCIENTIFIC EVIDENCE TO INDICATE THAT INHALING VERY SMALL DOSES OF MERCURY INCREASE THE INCIDENCE OF DISEASE OR CAUSE HIGHER MORTALITY RATES IN ANYONE INCLUDING DENTAL PERSONNEL WHO HAVE A MUCH GREATER EXPOSURE

SOURCE: JADA, Vol 106, April 1983.
TITLE: Safety of Dental Amalgam.
AUTHOR: Council on Dental Materials, Instruments and Equipment
Council on Dental Therapeutics.

STATEMENT: "Reinhardt et al (2) reported evidence of mercury vapor expired after restorative treatment. Mercury levels in expired air during removal of amalgam ranged from 160 ng/min to less than 40 ng/min and the level following amalgam replacement is about 10 ng/min for up to 200 minutes. No further measurement was made after this period. There is no recorded scientific evidence, of mercury vapor toxicity resulting from this level (10 ng/min) of mercury vapor. Further, none of these measured amounts of released mercury vapor have been documented as being associated with various diseases and/or medical conditions. Furthermore and it is most significant to note that there is no documented scientific evidence to suggest that dentists and dental office personnel who are exposed to much greater amounts of mercury vapor have a greater incidence of certain medical conditions or higher mortality rates as compared to the general population." (the terminology of ng/min means nanograms per minute and represents one billionth of a gram of elemental mercury. Each .100 milligram per cubic meter equals 12.5 nanograms of elemental mercury for each 10 second count).

FOR: Two references are cited in this portion of the ADA policy statement. The first is the work of Dr. Reinhardt and his associates who published in 1979 the preliminary findings of their research which involved the measurement of mercury vapor in expired breath after restorative treatment. The second reference refers to a study titled *"Mortality of Dentists, 1968 to 1972"* which was done by the Bureau of Economic Research and Statistics of the ADA and published in the JADA, Vol 90, January 1975. Both are excellent studies.

AGAINST: The ADA references the work of Dr. Reinhardt and his associates as proof of their position that the mercury vapor released from amalgam fillings is only a temporary phenomenon, and that the temporary detectable level is so low that it could not possibly contribute to or cause any problems with our health.

In a sense, the ADA is comparing apples and oranges and would have us believe that they are both the same. Dr. Reinhardt's work deals with determining the level of mercury vapor present during the process of removing and replacing an amalgam filling in a tooth. The purpose behind the experiment was to determine if procedures used by the dentist in performing work could minimize the patient's exposure to mercury vapor. The experiments were also intended to determine the length of time increased levels of mercury vapor would be present in the patient's breath after the work had been completed.

Dr. Reinhardt, in discussing his results, and those of his colleagues, states "The levels of mercury recorded in this study are low and quite transient. Consequently this study agrees with Frykholm's conclusion that mercury exposure occurring from the removal or insertion of amalgam restorations will not give rise to systemic mercury poisoning in dental patients." The paper concludes with the following sentence: "The significance of repeated exposure to small amounts of mercury vapor is not entirely understood, but consideration should be given to techniques that minimize exposure to both patients and dental personnel."

More importantly, Dr. Reinhardt states: "Statistical analysis was directed toward determining whether there was a difference between the amount of mercury vapor expired before and after the restorative procedure." What that statement means is that detectable levels of mercury were measured in the patients' mouths before anything was done and that this level only increased very slightly 200 minutes after the procedure of removing and installing a new amalgam filling had been completed. Citing Dr. Reinhardt's work immediately following Dr. Svares experiments in which he and his colleagues measured the expired breath of patients before and after chewing gum, leads the reader to the conclusion that they need not be very concerned with the results of Dr. Svare's work. Nothing could be further from the truth.

The results of the experiments related to mercury vapor levels after chewing were very dramatic. The work of Dr. Svare's group which was outlined in Argument 3 concludes with this statement: "It is thereby concluded that the possibility for significant mercury vapor exposure from dental amalgam in humans exists."

This leads us to the very positive statements made by the ADA concerning the lack of any scientific proof that low levels of mercury vapor from amalgam fillings are associated with any diseases or medical conditions and that mortality rates of dental personnel are no different that of the general population.

The key of course to the first part of the position is the phrase "scientific proof". This puts us face to face with the rigid scientific doctrine that precludes acceptance of "anecdotal" evidence as scientific proof. For example, you might have 500 cases on file that demonstrate that a particular disease or medical condition alleviated or was cured upon removal of amalgam fillings and their replacement with a non-metal composite. This could not be considered as valid scientific proof. What you would have to do to satisfy the scientific proof criteria is take those same 500 people, who had been helped by removal of their amalgam fillings, and put the amalgam fillings back into their teeth to see if the same disease or medical condition reappeared. Even with that, the results might be questioned because of psychological coniserations where it is possible to have a person get better or sicker by suggestion only.

This brings us to the heart of the problem which is dose-response relationships. How much of any poison or toxic substance must an individual take or what degree of exposure must the individual be subjected to before some clinical, identifiable symptom or sign develops? Consequently, it would be a straightforward experiment to take separate groups of animals and subject them to different levels of mercury vapor and record the resulting signs and symptoms. The animals could then be killed and dissected and the experiment would have shown what symptoms or signs the animals displayed at certain dose levels and what internal damage may have been done to cells, organs, glands, or body fluids. What experiments of this type cannot show is how much damage might occur from very small exposures over a period of years.

It is important that you fully understand the significance of this dose-response relationship. There are literally hundreds of scientific papers that show mercury can effect and cause some detectable damage to almost every component of the human body or comparable component of an animal body. However, there does not seem to be any way of proving or demonstrating in a human body that mercury is the sole cause of the detectable damage. To prove this in humans, we would have to be maintained in a totally sterile environment and not subjected to any other known toxic substance except mercury. This of course, is impossible. We are subjected to thousands of chemicals and pollutants in the course of our lifetime simply from the routine acts of eating and breathing.

Consequently it appears that for anyone to make categorical statements that there is absolutely no danger from mercury in amalgam fillings, they would have to compare apples to apples. By this I mean that you simply cannot lump the entire population into one grouping for any type of statistical analysis. To be correct, you would have to analyze that segment of the population who had no amalgam fillings as one group and analyze the remaining group with amalgam fillings as another segment of the population. To my knowledge, such studies have never been done.

When the ADA makes a positive statement that dental personnel have the same incidence of certain medical conditions and mortality rates as compared to the general population, it is a true statement of the facts available from existing data. What is not stated is the fact that like most of the general population to which it is being compared, most dentists have amalgam fillings in their mouths. Therefore should there by any statistical difference? The study cited by the ADA to support their statement on the comparability of dental personnel to the rest of the population, was only done on dentists. There have been no in depth studies done on diseases, medical conditions or mortality on any other personnel working in the dental office, that I have been able to find. Accordingly, I cannot understand how the ADA can make a positive statement concerning this segment of dental personnel. It is the dental assistants, who handle and mix the amalgam, that should really be studied, as that is when the greatest degree of exposure occurs.

What is required, at this point in our evolution, are epidemiological and mortality studies that will portray the incidence of specific diseases or the cause of death under three major sub-divisions of the population: those with amalgam fillings, those who have never had amalgam fillings, and those who have appliances or other devices installed that contain dissimilar metals. The results of such studies may well provide clues to many of the disease states or medical conditions which are presently identified as emanating from an unknown cause.

ARGUMENT 5
MEASUREMENT OF MERCURY CONTENT OF THE URINE IS A RELIABLE INDICATOR OF WHETHER AN INDIVIDUAL MAY SUFFER ANY BIOLOGICAL EFFECTS FROM EXPOSURE TO MERCURY

SOURCE: JADA, Vol 106, April 1983
TITLE: Safety of Dental Amalgams.
AUTHORS: Council on Dental Materials, Equipment and Instruments
Council on Dental Therapeutics
STATEMENT: "Studies, using radioactive mercury in amalgam restorations, have shown that the urinary excretion of tagged mercury increased 2.5 ug/1 on the 5th day after insertion of an amalgam restoration, and decreased to zero after seven or eight days. On removal of the restorations, the level of tagged mercury in urine increased to 5 ug/1 and then dropped to zero in two days. (4) Studies in humans (5-7) have repeatedly demonstrated and documented that biological effects, particularly central nervous system effects, are not manifested by the most sensitive neurological measurements until the human urinary mercury level reaches 500 ug/1. This level is 170 times the average urinary mercury excretion (3 ug/1) of the general public." NOTE:

The term ug/1 is scientific notation expressing micrograms per liter.

FOR: The ADA has cited four references to support their statement. The first (footnote 4) references the work of Dr. K. O. Frykholm which was a comprehensive study published as a separate issue supplement to the Swedish Journal, Acta Odontologica Scandinavica, Volume 15, 1957. Footnotes 5 and 6 refer to studies done by Langolf and his associates that were published in 1978 and 1979. Footnote 7 references a study by Miller and his associates published in 1975.

In Dr. Frykholm's study, silver amalgam containing radioactive mercury was inserted in the teeth of 5 male volunteer patients. After 7 days, the radioactive amalgam was removed and replaced with regular amalgam. The urine and feces excreted in 24 hours was collected every day during the 7 days the radioactive fillings were in place and for 7 days afterwards. Both the urine and feces were analyzed for mercury utilizing a Scintillation counter. The Langolf, et al. studies were to determine whether existing occupational hygiene controls were adequate to prevent neurotoxic effects in workers exposed to heavy metals, solvents and pesticides. The studies were done over a 6 year period. The researchers set up a series of tests for mercury exposed groups that measured the neurological functions of tremor, psychomotor performance, memory function, and nerve conduction. Each worker's level of mercury exposure was estimated by doing a monthly analysis of the amount of mercury in samples of their urine. A control level of 500 micrograms per liter of urine was established. Their results did indicate that if there were more than 500 micrograms of mercury present in the urine, the workers exhibited detectable changes in neuromuscular tremor power and in tremor frequency. However this level was not found to correlate well with short term memory loss. The work of Miller and his associates was similar in nature although they did not focus on specific urine mercury levels.

AGAINST: There has been a tremendous amount of controversy concerning the use of mercury urine levels as the diagnostic basis for determining toxic effects of exposure to mercury. I believe Goldwater and his associates said it best in their article published in 1964, "Mercury in the urine can no longer influence the living organism, since it has left the body. What it may have done in the course of its absorption, transport, metabolism and excretion is far more important." I think this really gets to the heart of the overall problem concerning the use of amalgam as a filling material. Don't tell me how much mercury my body is getting rid of. Tell me how much is still in my body, where it is, and what it is doing to me.

The controversy rages on even today although through the years there has been a great accumulation of scientific research that concludes that urinary levels of mercury have little or no diagnostic value: Fleishman, 1928; Goldwater, 1957; Noe, 1960; Meyer, 1961; Jacobs et al, 1964; Report of an International Committee: Maximum allowable concentrations of mercury, 1969; Siedlecki, 1971; Hibbard and Smith, 1972; Wallach, 1972; Cutright, 1973; Shofer, 1974; Eastmond and Holt, 1975; Yamaguchi et al, 1977, just to name a few.

From the technical standpoint, the procedures and instruments utilized for mercury analysis have undergone major changes over the years. The problem was considered critical enough that in 1978, the National Academy of Sciences published a comprehensive work titled "An Assessment of Mercury in the Environment" in which they included a 27 page Appendix on Mercury Analytical Methods. One of the points brought out in the Appendix is "Techniques for trace metal analyses have undergone considerable improvement in the past 10 years, leading to a need for assessment of earlier analyses." Another major point made was that unless the sample was "fixed" with certain acids, and stored in a proper container the loss of mercury from the sample to be analyzed could be significant. For example approximately 50% of the mercury in the sample could be lost in 1.5 days if proper procedures are not followed.

Scientists are continually discovering new factors that affect the amount of mercury that is excreted in the urine under various conditions of exposure. For example, Dr. Lie, et al. in 1982, showed that women had a higher mercury urine level than men and that in both sexes there was a reduction in urine mercury with increased age. Kristensen and Hansen in 1980 found that urinary mercury excretion patterns were greatly influenced by selenium levels. Other researchers have also shown that the amino acid cysteine has a bearing on mercury urine levels. I am sure there are many other constituents of our normal food intake that have either a negative or positive effect on our mercury excretion rates. Perhaps the National Acadamy of Sciences puts it in a better perspective when they state: "However, it should be emphasized that the current clinical limits for detecting the effects of methymercury in human populations should not be equated with threshold levels because other more subtle effects, such as behavioral or intellectual deficits, may not be detectable by the clinical procedures that were used." If you would like further proof as to the complexity of this problem, Cherian, et al. in a 1978 paper concluded that "urinary values are more likely to reflect kidney content of mercury".

In Dr. Frykholm's study cited by the ADA, there are some significant aspects that I feel should be pointed out. The first is that there was no evaluation of how much of the radioactive mercury (the amount originally placed in the tooth) was excreted and how much was retained in the body. In the study published by Dr. Cherian and his associates in 1978, which utilized radioactive mercury vapor, they indicate that it is very probable that radioactive mercury is exchanged with a substantial pool of non-radioactive mercury before entering the urine and that the probable location of this pool is the kidneys since the kidneys are the major organs of mercury accumulation in the body. They conclude their article by stating "we therefore have no satisfactory indicator media at this time to indicate brain concentrations of mercury vapor. A similar conclusion has been obtained from animal studies."

Another aspect of Dr. Frykholm's study that is quite significant is that the radioactive fillings were only in place for seven days and, although the radioactive mercury urine levels decreased to zero values on the seventh to eighth day, radioactive mercury was still being detected in the feces of the test patients until the 13th day. This tends to graphically illustrate that the transport and distribution of mercury in the human body is indeed a very complex matter, and critically involves it's biological half-life. In this regard, the material used in Dr. Frykholm's study had a half-life of 47 days. This should have taken over 141 days for the test patients to get rid of all the mercury inhaled during the test.

To insure that you fully understand the significance of this in relation to the overall problem of mercury vapor being released from amalgam fillings, the work of Cherian and his associates showed that the total cumulative amount of radioactive mercury contained in the urine and fecal excretion of their test patients amounted to approximately 11.6% of the retained dose. In this same context, Goodman and Gilman in their book, The Pharmacological Basis of Therapeutics, 6th edition 1980, also state: "Excretion of methylmercury in man is mainly in the feces; less than 10% of a dose appears in urine (Echman et al 1968). The biological half-life of methylmercury in man is about 65 days (Eckman et al, 1968; Bakir et al, 1973)." To make the problem more complex, Clarkson in 1972, in discussing an experiment that had been conducted on rats stated: "These findings suggest that rats exposed daily to mercury would gradually accumulate the metal throughout their life spans." Please bear the last point in mind at all times because I think what the research I have quoted says, is that all of the mercury doesn't come out of our bodies and that as long as we have a continuous source, our bodies will continue to accumulate mercury in almost every organ over our entire life span.

With regard to the work of Langolf et al, they are addressing an industrial exposure problem involving concentrations of mercury vapor in the work place. I cannot really take exception to their findings that there is a relationship between urine mercury levels greater than 500 micrograms per liter and manifestations of neurological damage.

However, not stated by the ADA, is another finding of the Langolf group which I consider to be more significant to the problem we all are concerned with. The results of their testing of short term memory showed a decrease in short term memory capacity and that these sub-clinical short term memory effects could occur at urinary mercury levels maintained consistently below the 500 microgram limit. They also concluded that these short term memory changes resemble those that occur with aging and state "In fact, the changes in memory function associated with an increase in twelve month average urinary mercury of only 100 micrograms per liter may be functionally comparable to the effects of 10 years of aging.''

Based on a comprehensive review of the literature, the prevailing view of most scientists and researchers is that the use of mercury urine levels as a valid and reliable indicator of potential damage to the human body is without merit. Future research efforts must concentrate on determining what damage is being done to our bodies by the mercury that isn't excreted in our urine, feces, breath or sweat, or in the milk of nursing mothers.

ARGUMENT 6
ONLY INDIVIDUALS SENSITIVE TO MERCURY SHOULD CONSIDER REPLACING THEIR AMALGAM FILLINGS

SOURCE: JADA, Vol 106, April 1983.
TITLE: Safety of Dental Amalgam.
AUTHOR: Council on Dental Materials, Instruments and Equipment
Council on Dental Therapeutics
STATEMENT: Two different statements are made. One in the body of the article and the other as the concluding paragraph. "The Association has previously cautioned that in extremely rare cases, individuals may develop either mercury sensitivity or an allergic reaction from contact with mercury. Patients, as well as dental office personnel, may be affected. Symptoms may vary from a local dermatitis near recently placed amalgam restorations to a generalized erythema over the entire body." (Dermatitis is defined as an inflammation of the skin. Erythema is defined as a flush or redness of the skin produced by congestion of the capillaries) "The Association wishes to emphasize that, except in an individual sensitive to mercury, there is no reason why a patient should seek at this time to have amalgam restorations (silver fillings) removed. Indeed, the effect of such a procedure and further restorative operations could be detrimental to the patient's oral health, including the unnecessary loss of teeth, and cannot be justified."
FOR: The ADA cites no scientific studies or references to support their position.
AGAINST: The simple act of reading those statements leaves

one with the impression that except for a very few individuals in the world, amalgam is completely safe. Chapter 7 of this book addresses the pathology or biological changes in the human body attributable to mercury toxicity so I won't address them at this time.

It is important to explore the subject of sensitivity and allergy to mercury. Dorland's Illustrated Medical Dictionary defines sensitivity as "the state or quality of being sensitive; often used to denote a state of abnormal responsiveness to stimulation, or of responding quickly and acutely"; and defines allergy as "a hypersensitive state acquired through exposure to a particular allergen, re-exposure bringing to light an altered capacity to react. Originally, the term denoted any altered reactivity, whether decreased or increased, but is now usually used to denote a hypersensitive state. Allergies may be classified as immediate and delayed." Dorland's goes on to define 21 different categories of allergies.

Of the 21 categories of allergy defined, we should be concerned with three of them in regard to amalgam fillings. The first is CONTACT ALLERGY, "hypersensitiveness marked by an eczematous reaction to contact between the epidermis and the allergen" (epidermis is the skin and eczematous means an inflammation of the skin that is usually identified by redness, itching, small bumps or elevations, weeping, oozing and crusting). The second category is DELAYED ALLERGY, "an allergic response which appears hours or days after application or absorption of an allergen; it includes contact dermatitis and bacterial allergy." The last category is LATENT ALLERGY, "allergy which is not manifested by symptoms but which may be detected by tests."

Based on the definitions, it doesn't appear that there would be much difference between sensitive or allergic. Both would provoke some type of reaction. What I don't understand is how the ADA can imply that there can be any reaction at all from contact with mercury once the amalgam is installed in a tooth. That is because in a special article printed in the American Dental Association News, dated January 2, 1984, the Association makes the following statement "When mercury is combined with metals used in dental amalgam, its toxic properties are made harmless." If that statement is true then I suppose we should consider mercury in the same category as some of the common foods we get allergies to such as milk, wheat and eggs. To do that though we would have to get the "harmless mercury" into our bodies some way. This begins to sound more like a good mystery novel plot because the ADA also maintains that the mercury doesn't come out of the amalgam filling. So how can we develop allergies to it????

If I were a dentist, I would be very concerned about what the Association has said in their policy statement. They have placed the burden of identifying which patients may be sensitive or allergic directly on the dentist *without providing any guidelines* or tests on how to identify them.

A search of the literature revealed that some of the first symptoms related to oral health that the body displays in reacting to mercury are: bleeding gums, loss of bone (loose teeth), metallic taste in the mouth, and foul breath. How many of you have ever had one or more of these symptoms, and gone to your dentist and had him, or her, say "It looks like you might be sensitive to the mercury in your amalgam fillings"? Instead we are usually given a pretty good dose of "guilt" therapy by the dentist inferring that it is all our fault because we haven't brushed properly, flossed properly, or eaten the proper foods, etc. etc. Those reasons may all be true, but it could also be very probable that we are having a reaction to the mercury in the amalgam fillings. An allergic reaction, which the ADA dismisses by simply having a policy that states "allergic reactions are extremely rare". Nowhere do they have anything published that tells the dentist if he observes such symptoms he should actively consider investigating the possibility that the patient may be having an allergic reaction to mercury or the amalgam itself or possibly one of the other metals in the amalgam. This in spite of the fact that there are evaluation methods, equipment, and tests available to assist the dentist in determining whether a patient may be allergic.

Throughout the documented history of medical and dental use of mercury there has been published evidence attesting to its potency as an allergen. In some few cases, the severity of the reaction has resulted in death. This is not intended to be a scare statement on my part, but merely a statement of fact. It is truly tragic that such events have occurred. My concern is with the fact that mercury is capable of provoking many serious reactions in the human body and that the established agencies, both governmental and private, have not seen fit to do serious research on the subject.

It is true that the ADA has published some research on this subject. One such article was published in the JADA, Vol 92, 1976. This study, done at the University of Texas Dental Branch at Houston, utilized dental students as test subjects and covered the time period from their entry as freshmen until graduation. There were 98 students starting the tests and 74 participants at the end of the test. The students were tested for a CONTACT allergic reaction by means of a patch test. The patch test involved placing a mixture of mercuric chloride and lanolin on a patch that was taped to the student's forearm and left in place for 48 hours. It was checked after 24 hours and the final diagnosis was made at the end of 48 hours when the patch was removed. At that time, a diagnosis was made as to whether or not there was a contact dermatitis reaction. If there was, it was classified as a positive reaction. In their freshman year, 5.2% of the volunteer students had a positive reaction. In their senior year, 10.8% had positive reactions. (It should be pointed out that these were dental students who, in the course of their studies were exposed to the procedure of mixing amalgam and had from 10 exposures in their freshman year to a cumulative total of 54 exposures in their senior year).

I must reemphasize the fact that only a diagnosis of contact allergy was made. No effort was made, nor was the testing protocol designed to determine, if any delayed or latent allergy occurred other than the skin manifestations under the patch. The important words in the definition of delayed allergy are "absorption of an allergen". In other words, we have no way of knowing if the students experienced any physical symptoms such as changes in blood pressure, pulse rate, heart rhythm, etc., because none of the participants were evaluated for these kinds of reactions. It is safe to assume that some of the mercuric chloride entered the body through the skin under the patch as this is a documented avenue of absorption. In fact, the latest technique utilized by the medical profession to administer some drugs is done in almost the same manner, ie. absorbed through the skin from a patch containing the drug which is placed on the skin.

Another finding of the researchers Drs. White and Brandt, who conducted the study, was that there was a discernable relationship in the number of positive reactions of the participants that were related to the age of the fillings. Only 3.8% of the students whose amalgam fillings had been in place five years or less tested positive whereas 6% of those whose amalgam fillings were more than five years old tested positive.

There had been a previous study, similar in nature, done by Djerassi and Berova in Sophia, Bulgaria which was published in the International Dental Journal in 1969. This study did not use dental students as test subjects. In fact, anyone who had been in contact with amalgam professionally was specifically excluded from participating in the study. The purpose of their study was to determine: "Whether it is possible that the sensitization from amalgam may be due exclusively to dental restorations; whether the time the amalgam restorations remain in the mouth plays an important part in the manifestation of the allergic reaction; which component of the amalgam plays the leading role in the allergic reaction; which of the factors such as age, sex, occupation, etc. of the patient favor sensitization by amalgam".

The study had 240 test subjects. Of this number, 180 had amalgam fillings and 60 had no amalgam restorations at all. The subjects were divided into 4 groups of 60 persons each according to the following categories:

1. Healthy; with amalgam restorations.
2. Sick (non-allergic diseases); with amalgam restorations.
3. Allergic patients; with amalgam restorations.
4. A control group; without amalgam restorations.

The subjects were then patch tested for allergic reactions not only to mercury, but to the amalgam itself, and each one of its component metals of silver, copper, tin and zinc. These results were read 24 and 48 hours after testing. Their results were much more startling than Drs. White and Brandt's results: 16.1% of the entire group of 180 people with amalgam fillings, exhibited a positive reaction to amalgam and its components. The positive reactions occurred within the groups as follows: 8.3% in healthy persons; 13.3% in non-allergic patients, and 26.6% in allergic patients. Exceptionally significant was the fact that THERE WERE NO POSITIVE REACTIONS IN THE CONTROL GROUP WHO HAD NO AMALGAM FILLINGS. Another major finding that differed significantly from the results of Drs. White and Brandt was the percentage of positive reactions in people with aged fillings: 5.8% in people with restorations less than 5 years old; and 22.52% in people with restorations that were older than 5 years. Another finding of great significance was the number of people who tested positive to the components of amalgam. These results were as follows:

Amalgam—16.1%
Mercury—11%
Copper—6%
Zinc—4%
Silver—3%
Tin—0%

Based on the overall results of their study the authors advanced the hypothesis that "Amalgam can cause the formation of several kinds of antibodies directed to the amalgam complex as a whole, as well as their individual components."

Why were the results of Djerassi and Berova's study ignored by the United States? At the very least, the study should have been duplicated in this country to confirm or deny the results. The fact that test participants without any amalgam fillings did not have any positive reactions should have been reason enough. In regard to the last point, I invite the ADA to tell me how the 60 people in the test did not have any reaction to mercury when they maintain that we get as much mercury out of our food as we could ever get from amalgam fillings!

Do you realize how many people we are talking about that may be having undiagnosed reactions to mercury amalgam in their teeth? There are no statistics that I have been able to find that indicate what percentage of the U.S. population have amalgam fillings in their teeth. For our example here let's be conservative and say 65%, (It is more probably 85 or 90%) and for a total population figure lets only use 200 million. Of that number 130 million (65%) would then have amalgam fillings. If we use the lowest figure from Drs. White and Brandt's study which was

2%, we would have a total of 2,600,000 people who could be allergic to mercury. If we use Djerassi and Berova's findings of 16.1%, there would be 20,930,000 people who could be allergic to the amalgam fillings in their teeth. Is that a significant number? The U.S. Center for Disease Control would consider that a National Epidemic requiring all available resources of the government to be marshalled to find a solution to the problem.

Although I'm not from Missouri, their "show me" attitude seems appropriate for the problem. It would appear to be a prudent action at this time for the National Institutes of Health through their Allergy and Dental Research divisions to set up a test protocol that would answer the question once and for all. That doesn't seem to be too unreasonable a request, especially when you consider some of the grants that have been made to study some really diverse subjects that serve no apparent useful purpose to mankind.

ARGUMENT 7
ONCE MERCURY IS COMBINED WITH OTHER METALS USED IN DENTAL AMALGAM ITS TOXIC PROPERTIES ARE MADE HARMLESS

SOURCE: American Dental Association News, Jan 2, 1984
TITLE: To the Dental Patient.
AUTHOR: American Dental Association.
STATEMENT: "Isn't mercury a poison? When mercury is combined with the metals used in dental amalgam, its toxic properties are made harmless. Moreover, the safety of dental amalgam has been studied for nearly a century, and all documented research indicates that, for the vast majority of dental patients, mercury-containing amalgams present no health hazard."
FOR: This statement is part of a fact sheet prepared by the ADA for dentists to give to any patient who questions the safety of dental amalgam. As the fact sheet was produced for general public consumption, no scientific references were given.
AGAINST: The statement is such a distortion of the truth that I was seriously tempted not to comment on it. However, to not do so would give the statement credibility, of which it has none. Here again, I can only conclude that the ADA is relying heavily

on the work of Dr. Frykholm as the basis of their statement, although I have no proof of that fact. In response to their statement, I challenge the ADA to provide documented scientific proof that even remotely provides any evidence in support of their claim.

Because the statement is taken out of context, and in all fairness to the ADA, I believe everyone reading this book should have the benefit of reading the fact sheet and accompanying editorial.

EDITORIAL

"The American Dental Association has been receiving an increasing number of inquiries from the media concerning the safety of mercury in dental amalgam. Subsequent information provided by our media reporting services tells us that these inquiries are being turned into news stories. Further, the geographical diversity of the news stories suggests that the safety of dental amalgam has become a nationwide issue.

Despite some sensationalized claims in the media that mercury in amalgam has caused a variety of maladies, no one has yet presented credible scientific evidence that properly placed amalgam restorations have been the cause of bodily disorders. In fact, the Association's Council on Dental Materials, Instruments, and Equipment recommends against removing sound restorations.

Still the media coverage may cause concern among your patients over amalgam restorations.

To help you provide accurate information to your patients on this issue, the ADA has prepared a fact sheet that appears below. We suggest that you cut it out and reproduce it for distribution for those patients who express concern.

If you don't need it now, keep it on file. You may need it later.

TO THE DENTAL PATIENT

Recent reports in the public media have raised questions as to the safety of dental amalgam. In order to provide you with accurate information on the use and safety of dental amalgam, the American Dental Association has prepared the following answers to the most commonly asked questions about dental amalgam.

WHAT IS DENTAL AMALGAM?

Dental amalgam is the material most often used to fill cavities caused by tooth decay. In general, one or more metals are combined with mercury to form a pliable mass. This material is then condensed in the cavity, which the dentist has cleared of decay. There, it hardens into a dental restoration or filling.

WHICH METALS ARE USED IN DENTAL AMALGAM?

Silver, copper, and tin are the metals commonly used in dental amalgam, sometimes in combination with zinc. Dental amalgam is used in about 75% of all single-tooth fillings.

DOES THE ADA HAVE AN ACCEPTANCE PROGRAM FOR DENTAL AMALGAMS?

Yes. To help dentists choose from among the various brands of dental amalgam on the market, the ADA has established an acceptance program to examine these products for safety and effectiveness. To date, more than 100 brands of dental amalgam have been accepted for the dentist's use.

WHY IS MERCURY USED IN DENTAL AMALGAM?

When combined with silver or other metals, the mercury produces a chemical reaction that causes the filling to harden after it has been placed in the cavity.

IS THIS SOMETHING NEW?

No. the basic technique has been used to restore decayed teeth for about 150 years.

ISN'T MERCURY A POISON?

When mercury is combined with the metals used in dental amalgam, its toxic properties are made harmless. Moreover, the safety of dental amalgam has been studied for nearly a century, and all documented research indicates that, for the vast majority of dental patients, mercury-containing amalgams present no health hazard. Mercury in small quantities is found naturally in the human system. And the average mercury level found in the general public is more than 100 times lower than the level at which harmful effects are usually reported.

AREN'T SOME PEOPLE ALLERGIC TO MERCURY?

In rare cases, a patient may experience an allergic reaction to mercury, usually in the form of dermatitis or skin rash. To guard against this very remote possibility, the ADA recommends that dentists maintain a complete medical history for each patient. If the patient is known to have such an allergy, the dentist may choose some other restorative material, something other than dental amalgam.

WHAT OTHER FILLING MATERIALS ARE AVAILABLE?

Gold is often used to fill teeth, either in pure form or alloyed with some metal or element other than mercury. Some manufacturers are working to produce composite resins (plastics), which soon may be available as acceptable alternatives to dental amalgam. To date, however, these materials have not proved durable enough to withstand the great pressure generated by chewing. Dental researchers are constantly seeking safe, new methods for restoring decayed teeth. For most patients, though, dental amalgam remains a safe and effective material for filling cavities.

WHAT IS THE "LIFE SPAN" OF A DENTAL AMALGAM?

On the average, amalgams serve for at least ten years, and very often they last considerably longer. Conditions in the mouth are constantly changing, and these changes affect dental materials and their function. Your fillings will last longer if you follow proper procedures for home care and receive regular dental checkups.

American Dental Association
211 East Chicago Avenue
Chicago, Illinois 60611

In closing the argument section of this book, I feel compelled to present further information regarding Dr. Frykholm's work not previously discussed. This is because I believe that his work must be considered as the greatest single factor contributing to the controversy we are confronted with today.

It is unfortunate for the population at large, that his testing protocol was designed as it was and that the better instrumentation and additional knowledge of urine testing subsequently available was not in place when Dr. Frykholm performed his experiments. His work, published in 1957, has been continuously cited since that time by every proponent of continued use of mercury amalgam as a dental restoration material. In effect, because no one seriously questioned his work, the findings of this one researcher have until recently contributed significantly to holding back progress, thereby, curtailing a concerted effort to find acceptable alternative dental filling materials. Why would any individual or corporation expend huge sums of money in research to develop a product to replace something that had been in use for 125 years, was considered safe, was easy to use, and above all was inexpensive.

The basis of Dr. Frykholm's experiments was to determine the extent of exposure to mercury vapor during dental treatment, both to the patient as well as dental personnel. This particular problem was selected because a review of the literature indicated such a study had not previously been done.

Some aspects of his study not discussed in previous arguments in this chapter are included now.

ABSORPTION FROM INHALED AIR: Eight human subjects were utilized and three to four amalgam fillings were to be installed in each patients mouth. Using a General Electric Instantaneous Mercury Vapor Detector, mercury content of the air within the mouth, over the fillings, near the mouths of the dentist and his assistant and in the room itself, was determined at one minute intervals. All of the test patients had previous amalgam fillings that were at least one year old. The results of this phase of the experiment can be summarized as: "Yes", some mercury vapor was present before the new fillings were installed, but this was around zero; and "Yes", the mercury vapor concentration increased during the installation of the amalgam filling. However, after rinsing the mouth and when the restorations had been covered with saliva, the recorded values were close to the ones recorded before the treatment began. Dr. Frykholm concludes this phase by stating that theoretically the most that exposed subjects, among those studied, could have taken up was about 0.1 milligram of mercury by inhalation and that this amount is far from sufficient to make the mercury uptake injurious.

Another aspect of this phase that seems totally unsatisfactory, is that no measurements were made after chewing and that the temperature measurements in the room were only 68 degrees Fahrenheit and the temperature in the patient's mouth was only 89.6 degrees Fahrenheit. Since mercury is more volatile with increased temperature and compression stress, it would seem reasonable to assume that a normal body temperature of 98.6 degrees Fahrenheit and the stress and frictional heat of chewing should have been considered as an essential part of the protocol. The latter statement is made with full knowledge and appreciation of the fact that Dr. Frykholm was only attempting to determine exposures during installation of new fillings.

There also has to be a question raised concerning the limitations of the measuring instrument used which could not detect mercury vapor levels that were lower than 10 micrograms and which used a 2 second sampling for the evaluation.. The instruments available today read mercury vapor levels as low as 1 microgram based on a 10 second exposure sampling.

Perhaps the most important aspect of this experiment is the statement that the levels of mercury vapor encountered could not possibly be considered injurious. That is a subjective judgment without scientific substantiation as no pathological evaluations were done and any previously published literature providing indications to the contrary were simply dismissed or merely mentioned in passing.

Some of the authors quoted by Frykholm who had published papers indicating a significant danger from mercury released from amalgam fillings were: Professor Stock in 1926, with subsequent articles through 1939; Toverud in 1932; Steffensen in 1934; and Hadenque in 1950. Publications after Dr. Frykholm's article was published in 1957 that have indicated findings and conclusions contrary to his were: Dr. Svare, et al. in 1980 who concluded their article with the statement "that the possibility for significant vapor exposure from dental amalgam exists"; Beste and Zoller in an article published in Dental Student, April 1976, stated that "elemental mercury vapor, in its final distribution, is found concentrated in the brain at levels 10 times those found elsewhere in the body."; and Bauer and First in their article published in the California Dental Association Journal, June 1982, state "even at low levels (mercury) can affect the motor control centers of the brain."

SALIVA EFFECTS: This was the 2nd area of experimentation conducted by Dr. Frykholm. There were two distinct aspects addressed. The first concerns the determination of whether saliva coating an amalgam filling stops the release of mercury vapor, and the 2nd deals with whether mercury is soluble in saliva.

The question of whether saliva coats the fillings and stops release of mercury was addressed during his first experiment involving the measurement of mercury vapor after a new amalgam filling had been installed. His statement on this is quoted as follows: "The protective effect of the saliva immediately coating the fillings after the insertion is completed, reduces the further vapor evolution to insignificant amounts." As previously pointed out, there is a serious question regarding the protocol used in arriving at this conclusion.

Contrary to Dr. Frykholm's conclusion the following authors published papers confirming little, if any, protection from release of mercury vapor is gained by a film of saliva over the amalgam: Stock, 1926 and 1939; Trakhtenberg 1969: Gay, et al, 1979; Svare, et al, 1981; Abraham, et al, 1984; and Utt, 1984.

With regard to the question of whether mercury is soluble in saliva, Dr. Frykholm concluded that silver amalgam is only slightly soluble. For you, the reader, the significance of whether mercury is soluble in saliva simply means that if the amalgam filling does release mercury compounds, they would dissolve in your saliva and then be absorbed in the mucous tissues of the mouth and gastrointestinal tract. It appears that here again there is a problem in the basic assumption from which the experiment proceeded. As part of his qualifying remarks relating to the saliva experiments, Dr. Frykholm states "It is well known that a silver amalgam filling which is already hard remains practically unchanged for many years as far as its volume, weight and shape are concerned.". Although the amount of research prior to 1957 appears sketchy, there were two reports that indicated finding mercury in saliva (which would also indicate that mercury compounds were being released from the amalgam filling thereby decreasing its volume and weight), Jensen and Dane in 1954 and Breguet in 1952. Subsequent research totally refutes any idea that a silver amalgam filling remains unchanged for many years.

Researchers have shown that a substantial loss of mercury occurs. This was proven by actually weighing the amalgam fillings in teeth that had been extracted. What these researchers found was an astonishing loss of as high as 84% of the original mercury content of the amalgam filling as shown in the following table:

PERCENT OF MERCURY CONTENT REMAINING IN OLD FILLINGS

Researcher	Year	% Remaining
Radics	1970	16 to 40%
Gasser	1972	16 to 40%
Gasser	1976	16 to 40%
Hanson	1982	16 to 43%
Pleva	1982	27% Average

What this means to anyone with amalgam fillings in their mouth should be obvious. Depending on the number of fillings in your mouth you could have swallowed or inhaled anywhere from 30 to 560 milligrams of mercury particles or vapor over the years. (Stofen, 1974).

REFERENCES

ARGUMENT 1

1. Safety of Dental Amalgam. Journal of the American Dental Association, Vol 106, pages 519–520, 1983.
2. Bauer, J. G. and First, H. A., The Toxicity of Mercury in Dental Amalgam. California Dental Association Journal, Vol 10, Pages 47–61, 1982.

ARGUMENT 2

1. Berlin, M. H., Nordberg, G. F., and Serenius, F. On the Site and Mechanism of Mercury Vapor Resorption in the Lung. Archives of Environmental Health, Vol 18, pages 42–50, 1969.
2. Kudsk, F. Nielson., Absorption of Mercury from the Respiratory Tract in Man. Acta Pharmacology Toxicology, Vol 23, Pages 250–258, 1965.
3. Clarkson, T. W., The Pharmacology of Mercury Compounds. Annual Review Pharmacology, Vol 12, pages 375–406, 1972.
4. Jernelov, A., Chapter 4, Conversion of Mercury Compounds in: Chemical Fallout, Miller, M. W. and Berg G. C. (Eds) Charles C. Thomas, Springfield Ill., 1969.
5. Abdulla, M., Arnesjo, B., and Ihse, I., Scandinavian Journal of Gastroenterology, Vol 8, page 565, 1973.
6. Edwards, T., and McBride, B. C., Nature (London) Vol 253, page 462, 1975.
7. Rowland, I. R., Grasso, P., and Davies, M. J., The Methylation of Mercuric Chloride by Human Intestinal Bacteria. Experientia, Vol 31, pages 1064–1065, 1975.
8. Heintze, V., Edwardson, S., Derand, R., and Birkhead, D., Methylation of Mercury from Dental Amalgam and Mercuric Chloride by Oral Streptococci In Vitro. Scandanavian Journal of Dental Research, Vol 91, Issue 2, pages 150–152, 1983.

ARGUMENT 3

1. Stofen, D. Dental Amalgam—A Poison In Our Mouth? Toxicology, Vol 2, pages 355–358, 1974.
2. Souder, W. and Sweeney, W. T., Is Mercury Poisonous in Dental Amalgam Restorations? The Dental Cosmos, Vol 73, Issue 12, pages 1145–1152, Dec 1931.
3. Frykholm, K. O., On Mercury From Dental Amalgam: Its Toxic and

Allergic Effects And Some Comments On Occupational Hygiene. Acta Odontologica Scandinavica, Vol 15, Suppl 22, pages 1–123, 1957.

4. Svare, C. W., Peterson, L. C., Reinhardt, J. W., Boyer, D. B., Frank, C. W., Gay, D. D., and Cox, R. D., The Effect of Dental Amalgams on Mercury Levels in Expired Air. Journal of Dental Research, Vol 60, Issue 9, pages 1668–1671, 1981.

5. Hursh, J. B., Clarkson, T. W., Cherian, M. B., Vostal, J., and Vander Mallie, R., Clearance of Mercury (Hg-197, Hg-203) Vapor Inhaled by Human Subjects. Archives Environmental Health, Vol 31, pages 302–309, 1976.

ARGUMENT 4

1. Reinhardt, J. W., Boyer, D. B., Gay, D. D., Cox, R. , Frank, C. W., and Svare, C. W., Mercury Vapor Expired After Restorative Treatment: Preliminary Study. Journal of Dental Research, Vol 58, Issue 1, page 2005, 1979.

ARGUMENT 5

1. Frykholm, K. O., (see No. 3 under Argument 3)

2. Langolf, G. D., et al. Prospective Study of Psychomotor Function and Urinary Mercury of Mercury Cell Chlor-Alkali Plant Workers. Rada. Toksikol Vol 30, page 275, 1979.

3. Langolf G. D., et al. Evaluation of Workers Exposed to Elemental Mercury Rada. Toksikol Vol 30, page 275, 1979.

3. Langolf G. D., et al. Evaluation of Workers Exposed to Elemental Mercury Using Quantitative Test of Tremor and Neuromuscular Function. American Industrial Hygiene Association Journal, Vol 39, page 976, 1978.

4. Miller, J. M., et al. Subclinical Psychomotor and Neuromuscular Changes in Workers Exposed to Inorganic Mercury. American Industrial Hygiene Association Journal, Vol 10, Page 725, 1976.

5. Noe, F. E., Chronic Mercurial Intoxication: A Review. Industrial Medicine and Surgery, Vol 29, pages 559–564, 1960.

6. Eastmond, C. J., and Holt, S., A Case Of Acute Mercury Vapor Poisoning. Postgraduate Medical Journal, Vol 51, pages 428–430, 1975.

7. Wallach, L., Aspiration Of Elemental Mercury: Evidence of Absorption Without Toxicity. New England Journal of Medicine, Vol 287, pages 178–179, 1972.

8. Kristensen, P., and Hansen J. C., Urinary And Fecal Excretion Of Selenium ($Na_2{}^{75}SeO_3$ and Mercury ${}^{203}HgCl_2$) Administered Separately and Simultaneously to Mice. Toxicology, Vol 16, pages 39–47, 1980.

9. Goldwater, L. J., The Toxicology of Inorganic Mercury. Annals of The New York Academy of Science, Vol 65, Issue 5, 1957.

10. Report Of An International Committee: Maximum Allowable Concentrations Of Mercury Compounds (MAC Values). Archives Environmental Health, Vol 19, pages 891–901, 1969.

11. Jacobs, M. B., Ladd, A. C., and Goldwater, L. J., Absorbtion And Excretion Of Mercury In Man VI Significance Of Mercury In Urine. Archives Environmental Health, Vol 9, pages 454–463, 1964.

12. Cutright, D. E., et al. Systemic Mercury Level Caused By Inhaling Mist During High Speed Grinding. Journal of Oral Medicine, Vol 28, Issue 4, pages 100–104, 1973.

13. National Academy of Science. An Assessment Of Mercury In The Environment. A Report Prepared By The Panel On Mercury Of The Coordinating Committee For Scientific And Technical Assessments Of Environmental Pollutants. National Research Council, National Academy of Science, 1978.

14. Lee, A., Gundersen, N., and Korsgaard, K.J., Mercury In Urine— Sex, Age and Geographic Differences In A Reference Population. Scandinavian Journal Work Environment Health, Vol 8, pages 129–133, 1982.

15. Cherian, M. G., Hursh, J. B., Clarkson, T. W., and Allen J., Radioactive Mercury Distribution In Biological Fluids and Excretion In Human Subjects After Inhalation Of Mercury Vapor. Archives Environmental Health, Vol 33, Issue 3, pages 109–114, 1978.

16. Clarkson, T. W., (See No. 3 of Argument 2)

17. Eckman, L., et al. Metabolism and Retention of Methyl—203—Mercury Nitrate in Man. Nordic Medicine, Vol 79, pages 450–456, 1968.

18. Goodman and Gillman's., The Pharmacological Basis of Therapeutics, 6th Ed, 1980. Macmillan Publishing Co., Inc., New York.

19. Bakir, F., et al. Methylmercury Poisoning in Iraq, An Interuniversity Report. Science, Vol 181, pages 230–241, 1973.

20. Langolf G. D., et al. Measurements of Neurological Functions in Evaluations of Exposure to Neurotoxic Agents. Annals of Occupational Hygiene, Vol 24, Issue 3, pages 293–296, 1981.

ARGUMENT 6

1. Dorland's Illustrated Medical Dictionary, 25th Edition, 1974. W. B. Saunders Co., Philadelphia.

2. White R. R., and Brant, R. L., Development of Mercury Hypersensitivity Among Dental Students. Journal of the American Dental Association, Vol 92, pages 1204–1207, 1976.

3. Djerassi, E., and Berova, N., The Possibilities of Allergic Reactions From Silver Amalgam Restorations. International Dental Journal, Vol 19, Issue 4, pages 481–488, 1969.

ARGUMENT 7

1. Stock, A., The Hazards of Mercury Vapor. Zeitschr Angew Chem, Vol 39, pages 461–488, 1926.

2. Toverud, G. Om "kvikksolvforgiftning" fra amalgam. Den Norske Tannlaegeforenings tidende, Vol 42: pages 181–191, 1932.

3. Steffensen, K., Om kronisk Kviksolvforgiftning foraarsaget af Tand-plomber. Ugeskr. laeger, Vol 96, pages 855–858, 1934.

4. Hadengue, A., et al. Note sur lelimination urinaire du mercure. Arch Mal Profess, Vol 11, pages 45–47, 1950.

5. Jensen, A. T., and Dano, M., Chrystallography of Dental Calculus and the Precipitation of Certain Calcium Phosphates. J Dent Res, Vol 33, pages 741–750, 1954.

6. Breguet, P., Action de la salive sur les amalgames dentaires. These. Geneve, 1952.

7. Abraham, J. E., et al. The effect of dental amalgam restorations on blood mercury. J Dent Res, Vol 63, Issue 1, pages 71–73, Jan 1984.

8. Utt, H. D., "Mercury breath" . . . How much is too much? Cal Dent Assoc J, pages 41–45, February 1984.

CHAPTER 5

DO WE REALLY HAVE ELECTRICITY IN OUR MOUTHS?

The answer is a strong "yes", if we have more than one kind of metal in our mouths. A weak "yes" if only one kind of metal is present. (Phillips, 1973) (Hyams et al, 1933) (Solomon, 1933) The answer is based in chemistry where all metals have been identified or graded by their electropotential. You may think that a piece of metal is a solid object that remains silent and unchanged forever. That is not the case at all. If that were true, then the metal in our cars would never corrode (rust). In chemistry, all metals have been classified by their electropotential from strong to weak. In one sense you might say that all metals are reservoirs of energy which are called electrons. The stronger the energy capability of the metal the more electrons it can attract. The weaker the energy force of the metal the easier it releases or gives up some of its electrons. This is so because electrons are always negative and always move from the weaker to the stronger attraction. Therefore, if you can get these electrons flowing through some kind of a conductor or transport medium, you will have an electrical current.

That last sentence is the key. The stronger energy source has to be connected in some way to the weaker energy source in order to have the electrons flow from one to the other. Aqueous solutions that have metal ions in them are called electrolytes and are capable of conducting or transporting an electrical current.

The aqueous solutions that don't have any metal ions are called nonelectrolytes. SO WHAT? What has all this got to do with me and my mouth?

Your saliva, which is an aqueous solution, is full of metal ions, particularly the life essential ones like sodium, potassium, calcium and magnesium, and also many others. This means that our saliva is an electrolyte. Now we have an electrolyte in our mouths bathing all our teeth and tissues with a film of liquid that has the capability of transporting or conducting electrical current from one point to another.

What else do we have in our mouths? Oxygen, which can cause metal to give up electrons by a process called oxidation (just like on your car when it starts to rust); strong and weak acids from our food and drinks, such as coffee, tea, colas, and citrus juices that can cause a chemical action to occur in the metals; friction caused from chewing which also generates heat; and temperature differences from the hot and cold food and drinks that we ingest. All of these are capable of exciting or generating activity in metal.

Where do we stand when we have metal in our teeth like amalgam, or gold, or chromium, or aluminum, etc.? What we have, is a potential electrical generating plant. Everything that's needed to cause electrons to flow from one point to another is present. We also have tissue composed of millions of cells that all have some of the electrolytes around them or inside of them. We also have nerves which, for our oversimplified description, can act as transmission lines carrying electric charges to other parts of the body.

Let's explore a common example of a gold crown and an amalgam filling next to it and see what can happen. The first thing we have to investigate is corrosion of the amalgam filling. Webster's Dictionary defines corrode as "1. to eat away gradually as if by gnawing, especially chemical action. 2. to impair or deteriorate." When an amalgam filling is installed in a tooth, it is subjected to all the chemicals we put in our mouths which are part of our normal intake of food and drink, and also to some of those produced by our own bodies. The acid or alkaline status of our saliva will vary with our food intake and individual body chemistry. All of this starts corroding or rusting away that amalgam as soon as it is installed. That's one reason why you periodically have to have amalgam fillings replaced. Maybe you have even had the experience of a filling becoming loose and falling out. I wonder how that happened? Although the ADA has stated (ADA News, Jan 2, 1984) that amalgam fillings last for 10 years, this is not a correct statement. Some will of course, but recent research (Smales and Gerke, et al. 1983) has shown that within 3 years, 13% of a group of 720 restorations had heavy surface tarnishing and all 720 already showed some signs of deterioration. Hamilton, et al. 1983, in a 10 year study reported that 35 of 99 amalgam restorations began showing deterioration at the end of the 1st year and that at the end of 10 years only 17% of the original molar restorations remained functional.

Besides the chemical corrosion in our mouths we also have the corrosion that can be caused by the electrical activity we previously discussed. We have both of these factors increasing the corrosion of the amalgam which, in the process, is releasing metal ions into our saliva. This corrosion may also reduce the strength of the filling and cause increased marginal breakdown of the amalgam. There are processes by which mercury (and other metals in the amalgam) is continually being released as vapor and abraded particles.

Let us return to our gold crown and amalgam filling example, and the possible problems (other than the release of mercury) caused by all the electrical activity in our mouths. Electrogalvanic activity associated with having metal in your mouth is not a new discovery or phenomenon. To the best of my knowledge, it was first discussed in scientific literature in 1878 by Dr. Henry S. Chase of St. Louis and Dr. S. B. Palmer of Syracuse N.Y. There have been a tremendous number of studies published since that date, all confirming the electrical discharge phenomonen associated with having metals in our mouths.

Is it significant? To answer that question I would like to quote from a 1933 article by Dr. Hyams and his associates published in the Canadian Medical Association Journal. Please keep in mind that this article was written fifty one (51) years ago:

"Lain, (3) Lippman, (4) Ullman and others have drawn attention to the fact that dissimilar metals in the oral cavity may be responsible for local objective changes such as acute and chronic inflammation, blanched or grayish patches, erosions, ulcers, areas of leukoplakia and pigmentation. Lain has numbered among the objective changes in the metallic dentures, discoloration, areas of erosion, disintegration, loosening of restorations, and maladjustment of dentures. According to him, the complaints which can be due to dissimilar metals in the mouth may include a metallic or salty taste, increased salivary secretion, burning tongue, dryness or tickling sensation in the throat, nerve shocks, nervous irritability and loss of weight. To these we can add, dyspnoea (difficulty in breathing) and diarrhoea. In both patients referred to above the original symptoms could be reproduced by restoring the original local conditions.

Sufficient evidence has now accumulated to indicate definitely that dissimilar metals in the oral cavity can be responsible for local lesions and local and general symptoms. It has been, and can be, shown that electro-galvanic discharges may be present in the oral cavity and the patient remain symptom-free. Perhaps some of the local changes, and, for that matter, general symptoms, can be explained upon a purely chemical basis. Certainly, as Solomon, Reinhardt, and Goodale (5) have shown, there is frequently no direct connection between the amount of current measured and the symptoms present. Recognizing the possibilities suggested by our two cases, it should also be appreciated that dissimilar metals in the mouth which are producing electrogalvanic discharges may be responsible for symptoms even in the absence of a local lesion or changes in the metallic denture present. Perhaps the nature of the patient's diet may be of some moment in such cases. We have tested many substances in solutions. To refer only to a few; when gold and aluminum are combined with milk as the electrolyte a current of 65 microamperes is registered; if an equal quantity of saliva is added to the same combination, 105 microamperes is generated. A weak salt solution under similar conditions registers 400, strong tea 110, zinc chloride mouth wash 300 microamperes.

The treatment is simple. The offending metals present should be replaced. Occasionally, destroying the contact between the dissimilar metal suffices. Before symptoms are attributed to dissimilar metals in the mouth all other important conditions must first be excluded. A milliammeter is inexpensive and easy to handle. Its use in office practice is recommended. It should certainly form part of the equipment of not only dental but also of large medical clinics. Prophylaxis is of course the chief consideration. When dental work is recommended and restorations become necessary, the use of inert metals, preferably noble metals, should always be urged.

If that isn't enough, more recent research has focused on "pain" that may be attributable to this source of electrical discharge. Many researchers have concluded that these electric potentials in the oral cavity may reach 900 millivolts or higher. The number 900 or higher becomes extremely important to us poor mortals when we take a look at the nerves in our bodies and how they transmit impulses to and from one point to another. Those of us outside the medical or scientific community, if asked to, would probably describe a nerve as one long continuous fiber connecting one point to another. We would be totally wrong. A nerve, for our purposes of illustration, can be considered as different lengths of fiber encased in a sheath. At the junction of each length of nerve fiber is a space called a "synapse". To get an impulse across this junction or synapse, it has to be fired electrically. Scientists have shown that the least possible voltage at which an impulse will fire across the synapse on a large nerve is 400 to 450 millivolts. When you think of this in relation to the fact that there are a great number of nerves in our bodies that make their way to the brain through a specific area of our jaws, the problem concerning the point I am making gets much easier to understand.

If a nerve happens to be close enough to a large metal restoration in our mouth that is capable of generating 900 millivolts or more, and the nerve only requires 400 to 450 millivolts to cause it to fire, we have all the ingredients necessary to cause "pain". If the metal in the tooth discharges its electrical current to the nerve, it will cause the nerve to fire and cause a nerve shock which our sensory system will then register as pain (it would be almost the same as sticking a pin or needle into our jaw).

The anatomic pathways pain may take from our upper jaws may explain why some changes can occur in reflexes, emotions, heart and lung functions. These pathways permit the pain to travel the network of nerves of the brain stem right to the hypothalmus and pituitary which are the control centers for our autonomic nervous system and major endocrine glands that produce hormones.

When we probe into repairing decay damage to a tooth by putting a simple amalgam filling in it, we have the potential of opening "Pandora's Box" with regard to the problems that may follow. To adapt President Kennedy's famous quotation to this situation we might well say to our dentist and to the ADA, "Ask not what we patients can do for you, but rather, what can you do for us to solve this problem".

REFERENCES

1. Phillips, R. W., (Editor) Skinner's Science of Dental Materials, 7th Ed, 1973. W. B. Saunders Co., Philadelphia.

2. Solomon, H. A., Reinhard, M. C., and Goodale, H. I., The Possibility of Precancerous Oral Lesions from Electrical Causes. Dental Digest, Vol 39, pages 142–144, April 1933.

3. Smales, R. J., and Gerke, D. C., Three-Year Clinical Evaluation of Four High-Copper Amalgam Alloys, IADR Abstracts, 1983.

4. Hamilton, J. C., et al. Marginal Fracture Not a Predictor of Longevity For Two Dental Amalgam Alloys: A Ten Year Study. Journal of Prosthetic Dentistry, Vol 50, Issue 2, pages 200–202, 1983.

5. Chase, H. S., Some Observations and Experiments Connected with Oral Electricity. American Journal of Dental Science, Vol 12, pages 18–23, 1878–1879.

6. Palmer, S. B., Dental Decay and Filling Materials Considered in Their Electrical Relations. American Journal of Dental Science, Vol 12, pages 105–111, 1878–1879.

7. Hyams, B. L., et al. Dissimilar Metals In The Mouth As A Possible Cause of Otherwise Unexplainable Symptoms. The Canadian Medical Journal, Vol 29, pages 488–491, Nov. 1933.

CHAPTER 6

MERCURY IN MY BODY?
WHERE DOES IT GO?
HOW LONG DOES IT STAY?

This and the following chapters in the book are the most difficult to write about in a form that the general public will be able to understand. The reason for this is that the real information you need to know can only come from highly technical and scientific research articles and books.

These are the real mystery stories of research and what science is all about. The dedication of the men and women who pursue these fields of endeavor make them the true unsung heroes of the the world's war for survival. Although only a few receive the recognition and acclaim they justly deserve. They all deserve and are entitled to our eternal gratitude and respect. Many devote entire lifetimes working to unravel one tiny facet of the greatest mystery in the universe, the human body. Without them, it would not be a very nice world to live in.

Thousands of research papers have been written that either directly or indirectly deal with the toxicity of mercury, and there is no end in sight. Nor should there be, until the scientific community knows, and understands, every nuance about this highly poisonous element. This includes determining exactly what it does in the human body, and perhaps of much more importance, how we can overcome its ill effects and limit future damage from dietary and environmental exposures.

Banning the use of mercury in dentistry and medicine is a

simple way to control some of our exposure. Although science cannot state categorically in all instances that mercury is the sole cause of some symptoms, syndromes or diseases, there are too many "coincidences" and correlations for it to be ignored or discarded. If mercury were the only substance available to combat various health conditions and sicknesses, nobody could fault the dentist or physician, who carefully weighs the potential harm against the possible good before making a decision for its use. Such is not the case. There is no life threatening situation that only mercury can overcome. There is no life threatening situation that requires your dentist to put amalgam fillings in your teeth; there are other suitable materials available.

Why the powers that be persist in their defense of this highly toxic, dangerous substance I will never know. I also cannot understand how we, the patients, have calmly accepted health professionals administering this poison to us, cloaked in the name of "Silver Amalgam", when we know it has the potential of causing irreparable damage to some of us.

As the title to the chapter indicated, there are three questions that we will try to provide some answers to in the following sections.

I.
MERCURY IN MY BODY?

In the previous chapters I have explained in some detail how mercury vapor is released by the dental amalgam. I have also discussed how we inhale this vapor and how we swallow or convert the particles that result from corrosion and abrasion of the amalgam.

Mercury from the dental filling can also travel down through the tooth into our bodies. Once the dentist has cleaned out the decay in the cavity, he prepares it for the filling material by first placing a liner and base into the cavity. This is a resin material that is supposed to seal the cavity and prevent any of the metals in the amalgam filling material from working their way into the pulp and subsequently down through the root into the bone and surrounding tissues.

The protective effectiveness of the seal is quite controversial. Early investigations claimed that they were effective and prevented any passage of the metals into the pulp. However, later studies using radioactive mercury amalgam fillings have shown, by tracing the radioactive mercury, that it does migrate into the pulp. Another study, done by O'Brien and Ryge in 1978, concluded that the sealer will only delay the entry of the mercury into the pulp. The pulp canal extends to the end of the root and has a restricted opening at the very end. This opening permits the body to provide blood and nutrients to the pulp (which is composed of tissue, blood, and nerves) and to the tooth, which in effect keeps the tooth "alive".

If mercury or any of the other metals in the amalgam get into the pulp, they then have a way of getting out of the tooth and into the alveolar bone and the surrounding tissues that support the teeth, where they can then easily migrate to other locations in the body.

Mercury is cytotoxic. This means it acts as a toxin or an antibody and has a specific poisonous effect on the cells. Bleeding gums and alveolar bone loss, which results in loosening of the teeth, are both classic signs of mercury toxicity. Of course these conditions can also be caused by germs or bacteria but according to Till in 1978, who used germ free animals in his experiment, mercury in amounts released from amalgam fillings could produce the same signs plus inflammation of the tissues surrounding a tooth. (This is sometimes called gingivitis, pyorrhea, or periodontitis).

Another very interesting entry route into the body was pointed out by Stock in 1935. He found that some of the mercury vapor coming from the dental amalgams entered the nose. There it was absorbed by the mucosa, and passed rapidly into the brain. It was found in the olfactory lobe and tract (where we have our sense of smell) and in the pituitary gland. A very intriguing study would be to see how many of the millions of people who have some degree of smell impairment also have amalgam fillings? Mats Hanson, a Swedish neurobiology researcher, and others in Sweden, have found that lead, thallium, viruses, and toxins are taken up by the nerve endings and transported to the brain and spinal cord by the "Axon Transport System". (This is a process of a nerve cell by which impulses travel away from the cell body). They are presently investigating their theory that mercury acts in the same manner.

II.
WHERE DOES IT GO?

Once inside the body, where does the mercury go? More importantly, I suppose, would be the question of how mercury moves around in our bodies. It travels by way of biological pathways. In effect, these pathways represent the "road maps" that provide routes for different substances to move along in getting from one point to another.

Scientists have established the fact that mercury has an affinity or attraction for thiols. A thiol is any organic compound containing a univalent radical called a sulfhydrl and identified by the symbol -SH (sulfur-hydrogen). What this really is saying, is that a thiol can attract one atom of mercury in the ionized form and have it combine with itself. It also means, because it is a radical, that it can enter into or go out of this combination without any change.

Amino acids are the building blocks from which the proteins of all organisms are built. The amino acid Cysteine has a sulfhydrl (-SH) as an integral part of its structure and can be found in both the interior and exterior of proteins. Cysteine is always contained in globular proteins and it is this protein that is involved in a tremendous number of functions in the body. Nearly all of our enzymes are made of globular protein and other globular proteins function to transport oxygen, nutrients, and inorganic ions in the blood. Globular proteins also serve as antibodies in our immune system, while others are in hormones or as components of membranes and ribosomes.

When we view the last statement in relation to the fact that cysteine, with its thiol (-SH) component, is a part of all globular proteins and that mercury is attracted to thiols, it is easy to see how mercury can move around in our bodies.

Some of the potential biological pathways for thiols to combine with the mercury ion are:

1. Tissue cell receptor sites. Whenever cysteine is present

on the exterior of a cell membrane, the potential exists for combining.

2. Hormones and Enzymes. All are proteins, so those with a readily accessible thiol group have the capability of combining with the mercury ion.

3. Erythrocytes. These are our red blood cells and they have a hemoglobin content which transports oxygen and iron. Hemoglobin contains 60 times as much thiol as does the human blood plasma. This fact gives it a high potential for combining with the mercury ion. In fact, anemia is frequently encountered in those individuals suffering from mercury intoxication. (anemia represents a reduction in the number of red blood cells contained in 100 milliliters of blood)

4. Glutathione. This is a protein having a specific combination of 3 amino acids, which is called a tripeptide. The important thing here is that one of the amino acids is cysteine with its thiol group and that glutathione is present in high concentrations in all cells. There is quite a bit of research going on at the present time, exploring glutathione and its functions, particularly in its role with selenium and mercury. Both of these metals can bind to the thiol group of glutathione. In fact, both are competing for the same binding sites. The difference being that when selenium combines with glutathione it becomes an essential component of several enzymes in the body, and when mercury binds to gluthathione it tends to inhibit or prevent these same enzymes from being formed.

One enzyme in particular that mercury affects is glutathione peroxidase. This enzyme is very important to us because it helps combat or neutralize certain substances (that are normal by-products of metabolism), that, if not controlled would destroy a great number of our cells. When our bodies are deficient in selenium it also means that there is less selenium available to compete with the mercury and, as a result, more mercury ions will bind with the glutathione. This can only serve to aggravate a bad situation.

Another very important discovery was that one of the enzymes necessary to make insulin work in our bodies is made from glutathione. In one form of diabetes, the body has plenty of insulin available, however, it doesn't seem to have any effect on controlling the blood sugar level. Some researchers are currently looking into the possibility that the presence of mercury combined with the enzyme prevents it from doing its normal job of making the insulin active. As you can see, the large amount of glutahathione available in our bodies provides a great thiol pathway for mercury.

5. Coenzyme 'A' and Succinyl Coenzyme 'A'. These are considered by some to be the most important enzymes in the human body and are intimately involved in the way the body converts (metabolizes) glucose (blood sugar) into energy. Because thiol groups are present, we also have the potential pathway for mercury. This, of course, could then have an impact on our energy levels because the mercury has the capability of disrupting or reducing the amount of energy we can produce from glucose.

6. Myosin. Myosin, which contains thiol groups, is the most abundant protein in our muscles. Together, with another protein called Actin, they are responsible for the contraction and relaxation of muscle. The importance of this is that with the thiol group present in our muscles, it then makes it possible for the mercury ion to also be present. The presence of mercury could possibly affect the normal sequence of contraction and relaxation, disturbing the rhythm and causing problems in muscle control. One of the side effects of this action could be tremors, which also happens to be a frequent symptom of mercury intoxication.

7. Cholinergic receptors in heart muscle. As we discussed in an earlier chapter, nerve impulses travel along segments of nerve fibers. To get from one segment of nerve to the next one, the impulse has to get across the synapse, or junction, of the two nerve endings. One group of nerves allows the impulse to "fire" across the junction through the use of a substance derived from choline which is called acetylcholine. Acetylcholine, in effect, becomes a bridge across the junction of the two nerves permitting the impulse to get across. However, every impulse that goes across the junction, uses up the acetylcholine that was in the junction. So before another impulse can get across, some more acetylcholine has to be manufactured and placed back in the junction. This requires a special enzyme which has a thiol group

as a part of it. Therefore, we are once again looking at a potential thiol/mercury pathway; only this time, it is involved with our nerve transmission system.

One way our heart muscles get nerve impulses transmitted to them, so that they can stay regulated, is through the cholinergic receptors (which also contain thiol groups) of the acetylcholine nerve system. So, anything that could inhibit or reduce the effectiveness of the enzyme that makes the acetylcholine, could also possibly affect our heart beat. Scientists know that the mercury ion can combine with the thiol group in the enzyme that makes acetylcholine and reduce the amounts available for insuring continuous uninterrupted transmission of nerve impulses.

Remember also, that the myosin in our heart muscles is responsible for contraction and relaxation dependent upon the nerve impulse received, and that this too, is where the mercury ion can cause a mixup of signals.

All three of these mechanisms, operating together, could possibly be the reason that an irregular heart beat is a frequently seen symptom in mercury toxicity.

8. Factor XIII. This is a protein that is involved in the processes of blood coagulation. As you can imagine, because of its coagulation function in our blood, Factor XIII is available throughout our entire body: outside our red blood cells in the plasma; inside our red blood cells, and also in the placenta. Factor XIII is normally not active and is only activated when there is a need to assist in controlling normal coagulation of the blood, wound healing, placental retention, etc. In its activated form it is designated as Factor XIIIa and in this form it is characterized as a thiol enzyme. This again means we have another potential mercury/thiol pathway.

There is some extremely exciting research being done regarding this compound. One recent paper demonstrated that mercuric ions can react with Factor XIIIa, resulting in inhibition of its activity. Because of this, there have been some theories advanced that it may possibly be involved in tumor growth and metastasis.

9. Thioredoxin. This is another protein in the body that has pairs of thiol (-SH) groups attached, which of course makes it

another potential mercury/thiol pathway. This particular protein is extremely important to us because it is intimately involved in the creation of DNA. DNA (deoxyribonucleic acid) is the carrier of all the genetic information of a cell. Without DNA, the cells could not reproduce exact copies of themselves. Researchers have shown that mercury, when combined with the thiol groups in thioredoxin, can cause an inhibition of the enzyme that results in its inactivation, which they have been unable to reverse.

I hope I haven't confused you by trying to explain in very abbreviated terms some of the most complex biochemical functions performed within our bodies. This is why we all owe such a debt of gratitude to those dedicated researchers who spend years and even lifetimes unraveling all these beautiful mysteries about how the most complicated processes of life really work.

Although we have only explained about the thiol groups, there are other compounds that mercury has an attraction or affinity for. These are chloride ions, amines, and amino acids. All of these in the right situations can combine with the mercury ion and each in their own way affect various body functions and processes.

The important issue for all of us to remember about the potential biological pathways is that they provide highways and routes that permit mercury to travel all over our bodies upsetting very delicate intricate life giving or sustaining functions, in the process. Don't let anyone tell you "there's no way in the world mercury can hurt you in the small doses that may come off your amalgam fillings".

III.
HOW LONG DOES IT STAY?

We have already touched on how it gets in and once it is in, what the different potential biochemical pathways are. Let's explore how it is distributed throughout the body and where it is usually stored or retained.

How, and where, mercury accumulates is a very complex problem that is influenced by many different factors. The degree of absorption is different for the various forms of mercury. For example, mercury vapor is almost completely absorbed into the body, whereas particles of elemental mercury that may be swallowed are poorly absorbed. The role of biotransformation and methylation must also be considered. Your diet, nutritional status, and biochemical individuality are all involved to a degree. For instance, if your diet is rich in foods containing Vitamin C, Cysteine, and Selenium, it is very possible that of the amount of mercury absorbed into the body you would accumulate much less than the person whose diet or body content is low or deficient of these particular nutrients.

Perhaps the most important aspect of where mercury will accumulate depends on the amount of binding material available within an organ or structure. By this I mean, that if the kidney tissues have a great number of thiols present at all times, then they have a built-in capability to accumulate a lot of mercury which has an affinity for thiols.

Consequently, as the mercury moves around the body in our blood and plasma, it will tend to accumulate in those locations that normally have large resident populations of thiols or other substances to which mercury is attracted.

Within the broad category of reactive sulfhydryls, scientists have also found that some have a greater affinity for mercury than others. Dependent upon the form of mercury, especially the forms such as mercury vapor and methylmercury that have the capability of readily passing through membranes, accumulation is going to be determined by the availability and degree of attraction to mercury contained in or at the host location.

Although the foregoing is a vast oversimplification of a tremendously complex problem and researchers are still trying to determine exactly how mercury is distributed to specific locations for which the above rationale does not seem to fully apply, they do know from their research where it accumulates.

The primary or target organs for accumulation of mercury are: kidneys, heart muscle, lungs, liver, brain, and red blood cells. Other storage areas or depots are the thyroid, pituitary, adrenals, spleen, testes, bone marrow, skeletal muscle and intestinal wall.

Some of the differences related to the form of mercury and its ability to accumulate in various locations or compartments are important. Elemental mercury vapor and organic mercury compounds possess the ability to pass through the blood/brain and placental barriers. Because of this ability to penetrate into the brain and placenta, mercury vapor and methylmercury (organic mercury) have the potential of causing the most serious toxic effects.

Mercury vapor also seems to have the ability to penetrate rapidly into all tissues, thereby giving it a fairly uniform distribution pattern. This same capability also results in initial accumulations in the brain that are very high in comparison to the uniform distribution elsewhere. Under normal excretion patterns, mercury vapor will tend to accumulate in the kidneys as it is released from other tissues. However, the brain level remains relatively high, because its release from this particular area has been shown to be very slow. In fact, there have been known cases where mercury retention in the brain has been shown to exist for 10 years or more after the last exposure. In one of those cases, the individual had only been exposed to mercury vapor one time. When he died 13 years after this single exposure, the autopsy revealed relatively high levels of mercury still present in his brain.

Although methylmercury also penetrates the blood/brain barrier its distribution between the brain, kidneys and blood seems to be more uniform. It also tends to have a greater distribution in the red blood cells rather than the plasma whereas mercury vapor will be more uniform in its distribution between red blood cells and plasma. Methylmercury seems to have a particular affinity for distribution and retention in the brain. Like mercury vapor, it too has extremely long retention times in the brain. Sugita in a 1978 paper reported brain retentions of 18–22 years for methylmercury.

A special relationship regarding mercury distribution exists between the mother and the fetus. Much higher levels of methylmercury have been reported in cord blood versus that contained in maternal blood. In animal experiments it has also been shown that there is a much higher accumulation of mercury in the fetal brain tissue than in the maternal brain tissue.

The overall question of retention and excretion is extremely difficult. Like everything else about the toxicity of mercury, scientists are continually discovering and publishing new findings. We could simply say that mercury has a half-life of X number of days, and leave it at that. If we did that, we would be obscuring a very important point.

Utilizing rats in their experiments, Rothstein and Hayes identified three different phases of excretion that have a significant role in retention and cumulative body burden. The first phase is rapid and depletes about 35% of the retained mercury from a single dose in a few days. The second phase is much slower, having a half-life of 30 days, which depletes another 50% of the originally retained dose. The last phase applies to the remaining 15% of the dose and has a half-life of approximately 100 days.

Dr. Clarkson in his 1972 paper expressed the opinion that the last phase would play an extremely important role in determining the total body burden that might be accumulated over time. Concluding that rats having some exposure to mercury on a daily basis would accumulate the metal throughout their life spans, continually adding to their total body burden.

It is apparent from that statement, that we should all be justifiably concerned with the potential for continuous daily exposures to mercury that may be related to our amalgam fillings.

REFERENCES

SECTION I

1. O'Brien, W. J., and Ryge, G., (Editors) An Outline of Dental Materials. W. B. Saunders Co., Philadelphia, 1978.
2. Till, T., Quecksilberabgabe aus Amalgamfullungen und Munddysbakterie als Ursache Parodontaler Abbauerscheinungen. Zahnartzl Welt, Vol 87, page 1076, 1978.
3. Stock, A., Naturwissenschaften, Vol 23, pages 453–456, 1935.

SECTION II

1. Lehninger, A. L., Principles of Biochemistry. Worth Publishers Inc., 1982.
2. Cooke, R. D., et al. Calcium and Thio Reactivity of Human Factor XIII. Biochemical Journal, Vol 141, Issue 3, pages 675–682, 1974.

3. Sarausa, M. M., et al. Human Factor XIII—Metal Ion Interactions. Journal of Biologic Chemistry, Vol 257, Issue 23, pages 14102–14108, 1982.

SECTION III

1. Sugita, M., The Biological Half-Time of Heavy Metals. The Existence of A Third and Slowest Component. International Archives of Occupational Health, Vol 41, page 25, 1978.

2. Rothstein, A., and Hayes, A. D., Journal of Pharmacology and Experimental Therapy, Vol 130, pages 166–176, 1960.

3. Clarkson, T. W., (See No. 3 Argument 2, Chapter 4).

CHAPTER 7

PATHOLOGY
DOES MERCURY CAUSE ANY CHANGES IN OUR TISSUES AND ORGANS?

The other chapters all lead to this one on Pathology. That is because it wouldn't matter how mercury got into the body, or where it went, or how long it stayed, if it didn't do any damage to our tissues and organs. Pathology is the branch of medicine that is concerned with any structural or functional changes in tissues and organs of the body that are caused by disease, or might in themselves cause a disease.

We keep calling mercury a toxic poison. It's now time to provide a definition of those two words. Dorland's Illustrated Medical Dictionary defines poison as "any substance which, when ingested, inhaled or absorbed, or when applied to, injected into or developed within the body, in relatively small amounts, by its chemical action may cause damage to structure or disturbance of function". Toxic is defined as "pertaining to, due to, or of the nature of a poison". When mercury is classified as toxic or a poison, it is pretty serious business because it means it has the potential to damage our tissues and organs and disturb their normal functions.

The subject is extremely complex, as I am sure you can easily imagine. So much so, that thousands of books and articles have been published on individual facets of each aspect of this branch of medicine. However, in relation to the total amount of information available on pathology, mercury comprises only a minor amount. Accordingly, this chapter can only hope to focus on some of the key pathological findings on mercury contained in the published literature. Please understand that I am not attempting to convey the idea that everything presented pertains to mercury amalgam fillings. However, it would be a disservice to anyone reading this book to NOT include critical information indicating the potential damage to the human body that mercury can cause, regardless of the source.

Notwithstanding all the latest scientific equipment and laboratory techniques, there is more that is not known about mercury's effects on the body, than is known. Each day, scientists and researchers all over the world are adding to the store of knowledge on the pathology of mercury and it's possible involvement in so many known diseases of unknown origin. That is why unraveling the mysteries of "Heavy Metal Toxicities" could be the greatest medical breakthrough since the beginning of time.

Each of the major areas of concern is outlined in the subsequent sections of this chapter.

I.
CENTRAL NERVOUS SYSTEM (CNS)/BRAIN

The central nervous system consists of the brain and spinal cord nervous systems.

The blood-brain barrier is described as an obstruction or a membrane (thin layer of tissue) which acts to separate the blood from the essential functional elements of the central nervous system. Its purpose is to regulate or filter the exchange of metabolic material between the brain and the blood. (Steinwell, 1961; Steinwell and Klatzo, 1966; Dorland's Medical Dictionary)

Without this barrier to filter the substances that otherwise might get in, the brain would be totally vulnerable to the thousands of man-made chemicals that we are routinely exposed to in our food, drink, and environment, and to those toxins produced within our own bodies.

Researchers have shown that mercury will penetrate the blood-brain barrier and enter the nerve cells from the blood. (Berlin and Ulberg, 1963; Ware, Chang and Burkholder, 1974).

These discoveries establish the potential for neurotoxic effects (poisonous or destructive to nerve tissue). With that as a background, let's look at some of the pertinent findings:

1. The blood-brain barrier is more than just a physical barrier. It also has a regulatory function by controlling the passage of selected biological substances from the blood to the nervous system. (Broman and Steinwall, 1967).

2. When less than one part per million (<1.0 ppm) of mercury ions are absorbed into the blood stream they can impair the blood-brain system within hours, permitting subsequent entry of substances contained in the plasma that would normally be barred or excluded. (Chang and Hartman, 1972; Ware, Chang and Burkholder, 1974).

3. Yoshino et al, in 1966 studied the biochemical changes in rat nervous systems resulting from mercury intoxication and concluded that poisoning by alkylmercury compounds might be the reason that he observed a selective inhibition of protein. Several other researchers doing independent studies confirmed Yoshino's observations that after mercury intoxication there is a great reduction of amino acids being incorporated into brain tissue. (Steinwall, 1969; Steinwall and Snyder, 1969; Cavanagh and Chen, 1971). The significance of this action was hypothesized to be an impairment of the blood-brain barrier.

4. All mercury compounds cause the same type of structural damage to the brain, but to different extents. (Chang, 1977; Schaumberger and Spencer, 1979; Gallagher and Lee, 1980).

5. Methylmercury produces rather complex changes in the metabolic responses of the brain, suggesting that the coordination of energy metabolism to functional activity (metabolic control) had been impaired. The alterations in intermediary metabolism in the brain occur at doses of methylmercury far below those producing overt toxicity in rats. (Bull and Lutkenhoff, 1975).

6. Human autopsy studies have revealed brain damage in persons who had been exposed to organic and inorganic mercury compounds. (Hay et al, 1963; Chang, 1980).

7. Neurological disturbances consisting mainly of mild tremor, ataxia (failure of muscular coordination and irregular movement), and sensory and visual loss were very prevelant in

the clinical observations of methylmercury poisoning. (Katsuki et al, 1957; Okinaka, 1964; Brown et al, 1967).

8. Gerstner and Huff in 1977 concluded that the symptoms of methylmercury poisoning are a reflection of damage to both the central nervous system and the peripheral nervous system. Rabenstein in 1978 stated that there was a latent period between exposure and the development of symptoms.

9. For long term exposure to mercury vapor, the organ that first exhibits functional disturbance appears to be the central nervous system. The toxic effects are produced after the body converts or transforms the elemental mercury vapor into mercuric ions. (Clarkson, 1968; Rothstein, 1971).

10. Progressive constriction of the visual fields, often progressing to blindness, has been reported repeatedly in almost all significant exposures of humans to methylmercury. (Hunter et al, 1940; Garman et al, 1975; Bakir et al, 1980).

11. Impaired hearing to complete deafness was detected in more than 33% of the affected adults and 50% of the affected children during the 1971 Iraqi epidemic of methylmercury poisoning. (Amin-Zaki et al, 1978).

12. Komulain and Tuomisto in 1981, utilizing rats for their experiments, found that methylmercury, even at low concentrations, inhibited the uptake in synaptic nerve endings in the brain of the neurotransmitters dopamine, noradrenaline, and serotonin. (A neurotransmitter is a compound secreted by a conducting cell of the nerve from its terminal which is bound by the next conducting cell and in this manner is carried along, transmitting a nerve impulse. Dopamine is a hormone like neutrotransmitter compound that is required as an intermediate step in the chemical process the body goes through to make noradrenaline. Noradrenaline is also called norepinephrine and is a hormone secreted by the conducting cell of the nerve that also acts as a neurotransmitter compound to the peripheral nerves and to some parts of the central nervous system. Serotonin is another nerve substance that acts to constrict blood vessels in many parts of the body including the central nervous system). In essence what the researchers are saying is that methlymercury prevented these neurohormones/transmitters from getting into

the central nervous system in the brain and performing their normal functions.

13. This last report appears to have a correlation to the information provided in 12 above. Parkinson's Disease is a degenerative disease of the central nervous system characterized by tremor, rigidity, hypokinesia (abnormally decreased mobility), ataxia (failure of muscle coordination), dysarthria (speech control impairment), and mental depression. The disease seems to be related to a depletion or impairment in the use of dopamine by those central nervous system neurons that require dopamine for activation. Ohlson and Hogstedt in 1981 studied six cases that had been diagnosed as having Parkinson's Disease and who had all been determined to have had exposure to mercury. The authors recommended further exploration of a possible association between exposure to mercury and Parkinson's Disease.

The studies related above and in the subsequent sections of this chapter, should only serve to reinforce the insidious nature of mercury and its ability to cause serious health problems. It can produce symptomatology that makes it extremely difficult, if not impossible for the clinician to clearly identify "it" as the primary causative factor.

We readily admit that live studies of the human brain and central nervous system present researchers with insurmountable problems. However, the ability to gain epidemiological data does not. There is an urgent and desperate need for investigative studies that separate and classify patients into two distinct categories; those with mercury amalgam fillings and those without. Studies of this type could help many people worldwide who are afflicted with health problems for which medical institutions can find no identifiable cause. Certainly it is not an unreasonable request to have these same institutions explore the mercury amalgam relationship through the simple collection of statistics on the living and those who die while under their care.

II.
RENAL FUNCTION

Renal and nephric are other medical terms used to identify the kidneys. These are the two organs in the body that have the function of filtering the blood. The kidneys are designed to filter out and excrete in the form of urine, the end-products of body metabolism. The kidneys also perform the important function of regulating the concentrations of hydrogen, sodium, potassium, phosphate and other ions in the extracellular body fluids (not inside the cell). These extracellular fluids include blood plasma, lymph, and cerebrospinal fluids.

There seems to be general agreement among researchers that mercury, which is also filtered and excreted by the kidneys, has the potential of causing serious injury to these vital organs:

1. Nephrotoxicity from mercury exposure is well documented in scientific literature: Friberg, 1959; Rodin and Crawson, 1962; Joselow, et al, 1967; Selye, 1970, and Wisniewska, et al, 1970; just to mention a few. (Nephrotoxic is defined as being destructive to kidney cells).

2. Pathological biochemical damage was found in the kidneys of various animals who had been exposed to mercury in concentrations below those levels presently considered as relatively safe for humans by the World Health Organization. Another significant fact was that the animals appeared outwardly healthy. (Nicholson et al, 1983).

3. Chronic exposure to mercury vapor may cause proteinuria (an excess of serum proteins in the urine, also called albuminuria) which may progress to a nephrotic syndrome. (Friberg et al, 1953; Kazantzis et al, 1962; Joselow and Goldwater, 1967). Dorland's Illustrated Medical Dictionary defines nephrotic syndrome as "a condition characterized by massive edema, heavy proteinura, hypoalbuminemia, and peculiar susceptibility to intercurrent infections". Intercurrent is defined as "breaking into and modifying the course of an already existing disease".

4. Kidney damage may result from excessive exposure to mercury as manifested by the nephrotic syndrome of edema, proteinuria, and the presence of cells in the urine. Such damage

may or may not be accompanied by an elevated mercury level in the urine. The nephrotic syndrome may be the only manifestation of mercury intoxication. In more severe cases of kidney damage, renal failure and oliguria may develop, leading to complete anuria. (Occupational Exposure to Inorganic Mercury, OSHA, 1973). (Oliguria is a condition where you are not excreting enough urine in relation to the amount of fluids you drink. Anuria is the condition where you are not excreting any urine).

III.
CARDIOVASCULAR

A recently published study by Abraham et al, 1984, demonstrated that mercury amalgam fillings can contribute to a higher level of mercury in the blood. It was felt that these increases resulted from inhaled mercury vapor reaching the blood via lung absorption. Two previous studies on this same subject failed to show any positive connection between amalgams and blood mercury levels. However, as in all studies dealing with human test subjects, results can be affected by a great many factors. In the study conducted by Abraham and his co-workers, they attempted to take a great many of these factors into consideration, which could be why their results were positive. Their results also correlated very well with another study done in 1982 by Kuntz et. al. that involved pregnant women and the measurement of maternal and cord blood mercury levels deemed attributable to amalgam fillings. (This study is discussed in greater detail in a subsequent section).

The real tragedy of this is not that mercury amalgam increases mercury blood levels, but rather that the true health hazards of this phenomenon have not been fully explored and documented by medical science. The potential of mercury to have a bearing on the genesis of our major health problems has been known for centuries yet its potential for subtle and insidious damage has never been fully examined and documented by medical science.

This is a round about way of saying that although some research has been done on the possible relationship of mercury to cardiovascular disease, it must be considered as extremely small in relation to the billions of dollars that have been expended and are continuing to be spent searching for reasons and cures for this No. 1 Killer. 3½ Billion Dollars was spent in 1981 on Heart By-Pass Surgery alone, which has nothing to do with finding the underlying cause that created the problem in the first place.

Some of the studies that have been done are reported here:

1. Mercury adversely affects the functioning of the heart. (Joselow, et al, 1972; Mantyla and Wright, 1976: Trakhtenberg, 1968).

2. Mercuric chloride blocked the vascular response to injections of norepinepherine and potassium chloride in rat mesenteric vascular beds (the large blood supply contained in the membranes attaching the small intestines to the back wall of the body). The mechanism of this action was related to a direct effect of mercury on blocking the entry of calcium ions into the cytoplasm (a site inside the cell where most of the chemical activities take place). (Oka, et al, 1979). Norepinpherine is normally released when the body detects low blood pressure. The nerves in the arterial muscles get the message and respond by contracting the muscle, increasing the blood pressure. Potassium and calcium are both involved in the process of muscular contraction.

3. Exposure to mercury compounds has been found to induce cardiovascular impairment. (Chang, 1977; Gerstner and Huff, 1977)

4. Myocardial infarction (this involves the death of cells and their coagulation in the muscular tissues of the heart, usually caused by a deficiency of blood due to a restriction in the flow of coronary arterial blood), coronary artery thromboarteritis (this is a collection of blood factors consisting of platelets and fibrin that bind with other cellular elements, some of which could be metal ions, to form a thrombus, which is similar to a clot, causing an obstruction to blood flow), coronary artery aneurysm (a weakening of the cell wall letting it push out forming a sac), AV Block (causing an interruption of the proper sequence of contraction of the chambers of the heart. The block means restricting the entrance of blood into the chambers), and premature ventricular contractions (early contraction of the lower heart

chamber) have been found in mucocutaneous lymph node syndrome (MLNS) patients. (Orlowski and Mercer, 1980; Adler et. al., 1982).

Some researchers of MLNS or Kawasaki Syndrome (Dr. Kawasaki first identified the syndrome) are attempting to find a relationship between mercury and the disease. Kawasaki was unable to confirm the presence of mercury in his patients and Orlowski and Mercer could not identify a source of mercury in their patients but did discover significant urinary excretion levels of mercury in six of their patients. It may surprise many of the readers to learn that this is not a syndrome that only affects people living in foreign countries. From 1971 to 1980, the Center For Disease Control (CDC) has received information about more than 400 cases of MLNS occurring in the United States. In a report in the Feb 25, 1983 issue of the Morbidity and Mortality Weekly Report, the CDC reported that since October 1982 there had been four outbreaks of Kawasaki Syndrome (MLNS) consisting of 43 cases in 4 states over a 3-month period. The CDC position is that there is no known cause for this syndrome. Coronary artery aneurysms are present in 17% to 31% of all the cases and the case-fatality ratio is 1%.

It is entirely possible that the signs and symptoms associated with this syndrome could be attributable to something other than mercury. However, based on the very limited amount of research accomplished that attempts to correlate mercury exposure to MLNS or KS, I am at a loss to understand how the hypothesis that mercury may be involved can be ignored without further exploration.

5. Electocardiographs (ECG's) were studied from 42 victims of organic mercurial poisoning. The ECG's were abnormal in all 42 cases. (Dahan and Orfaly, 1964).

6. A 1983 article by Carmignani, Finelli and Boscolo, reported a study utilizing mercury-exposed rats. They demonstrated that chronic exposure to inorganic mercury affects cardiovascular function by interfering with the blood pressure reflexes and/or the reactivity of catecholamines. (Catecholamines are adrenaline, also called epinephrine, dopamine, and norepinephrine, which are hormone like compounds that function as neurotransmitters). The effects of norepinephrine on

the alpha-adrenergic receptors of the cardiovascular system were significantly reduced. (Alpha-adrenergic receptors are thought to be located in the nerve fibers of the sympathetic nervous system. In this instance we are referring to their location in heart and arterial muscles where they have a direct effect on the amount of norepinephrine released in response to signals of low blood pressure. Norepinephrine would normally cause a contractile response in the arterial muscle to increase pressure.)

7. Clinical and experimental reports suggest that prolonged exposure to mercuric chloride increases sympathetic activity (Cheek, et al, 1959) and potentiates vascular response to epinephrine (Axelrod and Tomschick, 1958).

Epinephrine or adrenaline, as most of us know it, stimulates the sympathetic nervous system. It increases blood pressure, stimulates the heart muscle accelerating the heart rate and increases the blood output of the heart. Carmigani, et al, 1983, also investigated this potentiating vascular response of epinephrine that had been reported earlier. They suggested that the presence of the mercury ion reduces the amount of calcium available within the arterial muscle. Calcium is required for the contractile response of the arterial muscle and because there was a reduced amount available when the mercury ion was present, this would then cause the artery to open or dilate more than usual, resulting in a drop in blood pressure instead of the normal response to epinephrine which is an increase in blood pressure. Their conclusions also support the mercury/calcium findings of Oka, et al, reported in 2 above.

IV.
THE ENDOCRINE SYSTEM

The critical importance of the endocrine system warrants that we have some description of the overall system before we start discussing mercury's relationship to it.

Endocrine means to secrete inward or internally. Exocrine means just the opposite, to secrete outwardly through a duct. The endocrine system is composed of glands and other structures that have the capability to produce substances (hormones) and secrete or release them directly into the blood or lymph circulatory systems (lymph, derived from tissue fluids, is gathered from all parts of the body and returned to the blood through its own circulatory system). Once released into the blood, hormones have a specific effect on another organ or part of the body.

The organs or glands that have this endocrine capability are the pituitary, adrenals, thyroid and parathyroid, pancreas, gonads, the pineal body and the paraganglia (a collection of cells that can store and release the neurotransmitters epinephrine and norepinephrine).

The endocrine glands control or influence almost all body processes through the secretion of their hormones. The glands are under the direct or indirect control of the nervous system. When the receptors in the glands, or storage sites, receive appropriate signals from the nerves, the glands secrete their chemical substances in the blood which then function upon reaching their target organs or structures to maintain or restore metabolic balance. Hormones exert specific effects in the body on metabolism, growth, maturation, development and organ function. Hormones are generally produced as required, are inactivated as they are utilized, and are then excreted in the urine.

There are essentially three classes of hormones: steroid, peptide (protein), and amino acid. The steroid and peptide hormones have short half-lives varying from 5 minutes to 100 minutes, and circulate in the plasma. The short half-life usually means that the hormones have to exert their biological effects fairly rapidly. Factors controlling this are the availability of a receptor and an interaction between the hormone and the receptor. The other significant controlling factor is the amount or the circulating level of the hormone.

The steroid hormones are generally lipid soluble and bind to globulin proteins in the plasma for transport. The protein or polypeptide hormones are generally water soluble and circulate unbound in the plasma. The amino acid hormones have characteristics in-between the steroid and peptide and some have half-lives of up to a week. They can also attach to multiple binding proteins for transport in the plasma.

Anything that is introduced into the body that increases, or decreases, or affects the biological activity of these hormones can in turn cause the delicate balance control mechanisms of the body to go astray. The body cannot react properly which results in these imbalances causing such conditions as infantilism (too little growth hormone secreted), gigantism (too much growth hormone secreted), diabetes (too little insulin hormone secreted), to Hyperthyroidism (too much thyroxin hormone secreted). The extremes of some of these imbalances can be death unless, as in the case of diabetes, a synthetic hormone is available.

Now, let's look at some of the research findings in regard to the relationships of mercury to our endocrine glands and hormones:

1. The pituitary and thyroid glands in humans display an affinity for the accumulation of mercury. (Suzuki, et al, 1966; Kosta, et al, 1975).

2. The concentrations of mercury in the pituitary and thyroid glands were much higher than that found in the kidney, brain, or liver tissues in humans. (Kosta, et al, 1975).

3. Goldman and Blackburn in their 1978 article, describe experiments utilizing rats that were given mercuric chloride and radioactive iodine, the purpose being to determine whether the mercury affected the thyroid gland's ability to uptake iodine. (Iodine is an essential nutrient the thyroid utilizes in the production and secretion of its hormones). Rats given oral doses of mercuric chloride over a 90 day period displayed signs of mercury poisoning together with a reduction in uptake of the radioactive iodine. There was also a decrease in the secretion rate of thyroid hormones. After 90 additional days during which the rats had no exposure to mercury, the depression of thyroid function did not improve and was concluded to be permanent and irreversible.

Trakhtenberg (1974), in his experiments using radioactive iodine, showed there were significant increases in the uptake of the radioactive iodine by the thyroid even under low quantities of mercury. "Persons who show increased uptake of the isotope, as a rule, show symptoms of thyroid gland enlargement, finger tremors, emotional sensitivity, etc." As one of his conclusions Trakhtenberg states, "low mercury concentrations produce hormonal shifts and thyroid dysfunction." This was also found to be true with the pituitary and adrenal glands.

5. Animals poisoned with methylmercury exhibit stress intolerance and decreased sexual activity, suggesting both adrenal and testicular dysfunction. The data indicated impairment of the adrenal and testicular steroid hormone secretions. The authors concluded that the tissue levels of methylmercury required to cause the observed endocrine abnormalities of the adrenals and testes might be somewhat lower than those associated with overt neurological dysfunction. (Burton and Meikle, 1980)

6. Burton's study, outlined above, confirmed previous findings of Khera in 1973 and Stoewsand, et al, in 1971, that methylmercury diminished sexual activity in birds and mammals.

7. Methylmercury intoxication causes subnormal fertility and spermatogenesis (the process of formation of the sperm) in rats. (Lee and Dixon, 1975; Thaxton and Parkhurst, 1973)

8. Methylmercury intoxication causes impaired growth in rats. Diamond and Sleight, 1972; Kojima and Fujita, 1973)

9. Alomar et al, in 1983 related a case involving a 52 year old farmer who was diagnosed as having contact dermatitis and Addison's disease, attributable to mercury in the soap he was using. Addison's disease is due to reduced function of the adrenal glands and is usually fatal. Some of the symptoms are progressive anemia, low blood pressure, diarrhea and digestive disturbances.

It is evident from the limited information available that mercury has the potential of upsetting our delicate hormonal balance, either through increasing/decreasing the quantities secreted or decreasing the biological activity of the hormone itself.

If, in our wildest imagination, there exists the remote possibility that mercury, induced into our bodies from dental amalgam has the potential to affect our endocrine system, then some positive action is required. It is imperative that persons, institutions, and governmental agencies, who are involved in the decision making that dictate the continued use of mercury amalgam for dental restorations provide adequate scientific proof to support any claim that amalgam is harmless. As a minimum, the following actions should be taken:

1. Adequate priorities and funding must be provided for medical scientists to fully explore and reach a documented decision that either refutes or supports the claim of amalgam's harmlessness.

2. The opposition to finding the truth must be stilled. We can no longer accept 150 years of continued use as "prima facie evidence" that amalgam is harmless. As a part of this effort, a public apology should be issued to those dentists who made their decision to stop using amalgam based on available scientific evidence. These individuals have been placed in professional jeopardy by those opposed to finding the scientifically correct answer.

To those of you who have such a dentist, count your blessings. You have a dedicated health care provider who is more interested in your personal health and well being than he is in the orthodoxy of the establishment or the peer pressure that ensues.

V.
THE IMMUNE SYSTEM

Immunology is perhaps the most complicated of all the biomedical sciences. It becomes more complicated each year as researchers discover more about the immune system and its interdependence with so many other systems, organs, and functions of the body which previously had been thought to be unrelated.

The development of sophisticated laboratory equipment and techniques has permitted researchers to explore and learn more about our immune system. More knowledge has been gained in the last 20 years than everything that had been previously learned since the beginning of time. One important fact that is emerging from all of this newer research is that the immune system may be involved in the pathogenesis of all diseases.

For you to be able to understand the nature of the possible relationships that mercury has to our immune system, it is necessary that you have a general idea of how the system works.

There is a general principle underlying the living organism's ability to survive which is called homeostasis. It can be described as a state of stability, or remaining always the same, or being in balance. We endure from conception to death because of this principle.

For every action that takes place within our bodies, there is a balancing action that takes place to maintain homeostasis. For example, cells that make up our skin are constantly dying, but for every cell that dies, the body makes a new one to replace it. Every time your heart muscle contracts to push blood out into your arteries and veins, there is an opposite action that makes the same muscle relax to permit more blood to enter the chamber.

The immune system works in the same manner. For every foreign bacteria or germ cell that gets into our body, we are supposed to have a defense cell available to neutralize or destroy it. For every stimulus that is given for a defender cell to destroy an invader, there must be a counter stimulus to stop sending more defender cells. For every foreign invader that is destroyed, there must be some way to remove it from the body. For every one of the defense cells that is used up in the fight, a new one must be produced to be available for the next battle.

For every action there has to be an interaction and counter action. All of this is accomplished by a communications network that is so sophisticated and complex that science has only been able to unravel part of it.

What are the components of our complicated immune system and how do they function in the never-ending battle to protect or defend us? There are two major body environments in which the system must be able to operate. In the first is on the inside and on the outside surface of the cell. This is called Cellular Immunity. The second is in the fluids of our body, such as the blood, lymph, saliva, tears, and in the secretions of the mucous membranes in our nose, vaginal tract, and small intestine. This is called humoral (fluid) immunity.

Most of us are familiar with the two major classifications of cells (red blood cells and white blood cells) found in blood. Within the white blood cell classification (also called leukocytes) we have one type of cell that is the central cell in our immunity system. These are called lymphocytes.

There are two types of lymphocytes designated as T lymphocytes or B lymphocytes. These are usually referred to simply as T cells and B cells. T cells get their name from the fact that they are either produced in the Thymus Gland or their development is influenced by the Thymus Gland. B cells are named after bone marrow because it is thought to be the site where they are produced.

Both T cells and B cells have specific functions to perform in our immune system.

T cells are responsible for a great number of the functions involved in cellular immunity. To do this they are endowed with special qualities that permit them to migrate or travel to the site of infection or problem and once there to be able to independently move through tissue and capillary walls. They also function to defend against certain microorganisms such as disease producing bacteria that may get inside cells, fungi, poxviruses like small pox, and are supposed to provide antitumor immunity.

B cells, and their offspring the plasma cells, are responsible for humoral immunity. To accomplish this, the B cells produce certain proteins that circulate in the plasma. These are called antibodies or immunoglobulins. The immunoglobulins are the protein molecules that are possessed of the antibody capability. It is this antibody capability that makes the system so unique. Regardless of the number of different foreign microorganisms, the system can produce an antibody specifically tailored to attack every one of them.

The foreign substances that get into the body are called antigens. They are so named because they cause the system to produce an antibody so precise that it can only recognize one particular antigen. This is an amazing and extraordinary capability that the immune system possesses. There are literally millions of different antigens that your body may be exposed to, yet the immune system has the capability of producing a specific antibody for each antigen. Although we won't elaborate on it, there are 5 classes of immunoglobulins. Each class is identified by a letter suffix that relates to its specific biological properties and capabilities: IgA, IgD, IgE, IgG and IgM.

Let's look at an example of how it all works together.

Each germ has its own antigen. When one of them gets into the body, the body has the capability to differentiate between its own cells and a foreign cell. So, when the body senses the intruder, it starts the sequence of actions in motion that will neutralize or destroy the invader. The T cell recognizes the germ, or carrier of the antigen, and sends a stimulating message to the B cell, which then recognizes the antigen fraction of the germ. The B cell then tells the immunoglobulin to produce the specific antibody for the antigen. The B cell, with its antibody and with help from a special class of T cell (called a helper cell), surrounds, or engulfs, the antigen and neutralizes or destroys it and in the process also kills the germ. Once the job is completed, another type of T cell (called a suppressor cell) gets a stimulating message and proceeds to suppress further production, and eliminate most of the unused antibody. Some of the antibody remains alive, and in the blood, so that if the specific antigen ever returns there will be a built in immunity to it. The used up B cells, with immunoglobulin and dead germs, are then passed along to the liver and kidneys where they are excreted in the urine and feces.

The same sequence of events usually takes place when we have an allergic reaction. Except that in the case of allergic reactions, the type of B cell immunoglobulin antibody that normally responds is IgE, which has the capability to cause the body's cells at the site of invasion or contact to release histamine. Histamines are what cause the red, or flushed, skin reaction that is evoked when an allergic person is exposed to an allergen. This is why antihistamine drugs are sometimes effective in controlling allergic reactions. Allergen is another term used to describe any antigen that stimulates IgE production.

Now that background information on the immune system has been provided, I will list some of the reported relationships between mercury and leukocytes and the immune response.

1. High frequencies of chromosomal aberrations were observed in cultured lymphocytes from humans that had been exposed to mercury. (Vershaeve, et al, 1976; Popescu, et al, 1979; Skerfving, et al, 1970, 1974).

A chromosome is that portion of the cell containing a thread of DNA which contains many genes and functions to store and transmit genetic information. It is in this manner that lymphocytes are able to reproduce clones or exact duplicates of themselves. Aberration means that there is an alteration of the genetic information when it is transferred; it could mean the duplication, loss, exchange or alteration in the sequence of the genetic material which ordinarily would be reproduced as an exact duplicate of the original sequence. Any aberration of the chromosome constitutes a biological change that is thought to be one of the earliest actions leading to decreased immunity and increased susceptibility to disease.

2. The toxic effects of methyl and ethyl mercury on white blood cells included chromosomal breakage, alteration of mitosis (replication of chromosomes), and death of cells. (Fiskesjo, 1970)

3. Lymphocytes from mercury-diseased rats showed a significant decrease in their ability to stimulate chromosomal replication compared with lymphocytes from control animals (no exposure to mercury).

Mercury-induced anti-nuclear antibodies (specific to the nucleus or core of leukocyte cells in the blood and tissues) were found in more than 90% of the experimental animals.

Thymus and spleen lymphocytes from mercury diseased animals produced a migration inhibitory factor reducing the ability of the lymphocytes to travel to other locations in the body. This was determined by incubating the lymphocytes with the two antigens utilized in the test. Lymphocytes from control animals, not exposed to mercury, did not produce the migration inhibition factor.

A relative loss of suppressor T-cell function was found in rats with mercury-induced immune complex glomerulopathy. (a disease of that section of the kidneys called the glomeruli which is composed of blood vessels). Administration of low doses of inorganic mercury over a prolonged period induces an immune complex glomerulopathy in experimental animals. (Weening et al, 1980).

4. Mercury suppresses the primary humoral (antibody) immune response. (Blakley, et al, 1980; Koller, 1973, 1975 and Koller, et al, 1980).

5. Experiments were performed in the laboratory utilizing lymphocytes from individuals who showed no prior evidence of allergy to mercury, and lymphocytes from individuals who had known allergies to mercury. When mercuric chloride was added

to both cultures of lymphocytes, there was a transformation of the blast cells (immature cells) in both groups. The organic mercurial compound Merbromin (you know it as mercurochrome) also caused blast cell transformation, but Thimerosal (merthiolate) did not, even though it was determined to be cytotoxic (having the effect of a toxin or antibody that has a specific toxic action upon cells of special organs) (Schopf, et al, 1967; Caron, et al, 1970).

6. In a recent article published in the May issue of the Journal of Prosthetic Dentistry, Dr. David W. Eggleston, describes experiments involving three patients that demonstrated the ability of dental amalgam and dental nickel alloys to adversely affect the quantity of T-lymphocytes. In his experiments, Dr. Eggleston measured the T-lymphocyte percent of total lymphocytes in the patients' blood before and after the insertion and removal of dental amalgam and nickel-base alloys. In the first patient removal of six amalgam fillings resulted in a 55.3% increase in the number of T-lymphocytes. Reinsertion of four amalgam restorations resulted in a decrease in the T-lymphocyte count of 24.7%. Similar changes were obtained on the other two patients. Dr. Eggleston concludes by stating "Further research may determine the frequency and magnitude of T-lymphocyte reduction and alteration by dental materials."

There are a great number of other papers demonstrating the impact that mercury can have on our immune response and potential allergic reactions. The studies cited above adequately make the point that mercury can be a potent antigen and allergen as well as possessing the capability to alter our body's basic defense mechanisms to infection and disease. The implications of Dr. Eggleston's work provides additional urgency to reclassify the population into those with metal fillings, those without fillings and those with non-metal fillings. All future medical studies must consider this fact when attempting to determine the cause of disease in the human body.

VI.
ORAL CAVITY

The oral cavity could be utilized to make a great TV commercial advertising the outstanding health benefits available from the use of mercury. This of course is said with tongue in-cheek and bleeding gums. If you don't believe me just look at some of the benefits listed in the literature:

1. Mercury poisoning may be acute or chronic, but the systemic (affecting the body as a whole) reactions in the acute form are so serious that the oral features need not be considered. Chronic mercurialism (mercury poisoning) occurs after prolonged contact with mercurial compounds in a variety of situations, including therapeutic use of these compounds and as an occupational hazard.

The oral cavity suffers seriously in mercurialism and evidences numerous characteristic signs and symptoms (but they are not necessarily ones that can always be used to make a diagnosis of mercurialism). There is an increased flow of saliva and a metallic taste in the mouth. The salivary glands may be swollen, and the tongue is sometimes enlarged and painful. Hyperemia (excess of blood) and swelling of the gingiva (gums) are occasionally seen. The oral mucosa (mucous membranes) is prone to ulcerations on the gingiva, palate (the roof of the mouth) and tongue. In severe cases, pigmentation of the gingiva may occur. Loosening of the teeth, even leading to exfoliation (falling out), has been reported.

A toxic reaction from absorption of mercury in dental amalgam has been reported on a number of occasions. Frykholm (1957), after a thorough review of the literature and numerous studies on the absorption and excretion of mercury, concluded that the amount of estimated exposure to mercury from dental amalgam is not sufficient to cause mercury poisoning in the conventional sense. Nevertheless, this exposure may suffice to bring about allergic manifestations in patients sensitive to mercury. (Shafer et al, 1974, A Textbook of Oral Pathology) I bet you didn't think they taught about mercury in dental school.

2. Poisoning from the inhalation of mercury vapors is characterized by metallic taste, stomatitis (inflammation of the oral

mucosa), foul breath, gingivitis (inflammation of the gum tissue), and excessive salivation. Necrosis (death of the tissue) of the alveolar processes (the bony sockets in which the roots of the teeth are attached), loosening of the teeth, and discoloration of the gingival margins may appear later. (Goodman and Gillman's, The Pharmacological Basis of Therapeutics, 1980)

3. Two cases of Multiple Polypous Hyperplasias (growths, polyps, protruding from the mucous membrane that result from an abnormal increase of normal cells in normal arrangement in the tissue) of the oral mucosa that disappeared after removal of the amalgam fillings. Both patients had diseased lymph nodes in the neck. Metal ions were found in the biopsied tissues. (Bergenholtz, 1965)

4. Local inflammatory reactions induced by amalgam fillings have been observed in the gingival tissue. (Zander, 1957; App, 1961; Freden, et al, 1974).

5. Mercury levels of over 1200 micrograms per gram of tissue were found at the root tips of teeth having both gold and amalgam restorations. Up to a few hundred micrograms per gram of tissue were found at the root tips of those teeth having only amalgam restorations. The levels recorded increased with time and did not come from food. (Till and Maly, 1978).

I apologize for my opening remarks in this section. It certainly isn't a joking matter.

The information cited above, provides substantiation that the mercury can migrate out of the amalgam, as well as evidence of its potential toxicity. The point of departure between the believers and non-believers is the statement by Frykholm "the estimated exposure to mercury from dental amalgam is not sufficient to cause mercury poisoning in the conventional sense". This same philosophy is essentially embraced by the ADA and responsible government agencies. The fallacy of the philosophy is that it cannot be substantiated by scientific proof because sufficient research on the pathology and biochemistry of micro doses of mercury (micromercurialism) has not been done. In fact, there is not even a definition of the word micromercurialism contained in the medical dictionaries that I checked. In their minds, the condition doesn't even exist.

VII.
MERCURY TOXICITY IN THE HUMAN REPRODUCTIVE CYCLE
MOTHER? EMBRYO? FETUS? INFANT?

There appears to be an ever increasing number of children born who are either mentally or physically impaired, or both. Medical science is conducting some investigations into the phenomenon in relation to some of the more prevalent diseases that are manifested in the newborn. However, it is certainly an area of exploration worthy of a major national effort.

From the time of fertilization until birth, the offspring is dependent upon the mother for all sources of nutrition, as well as for routes of elimination for metabolic wastes. There are essentially four major areas that are considered to be critical or determining, in the outcome of fetal development: 1. The mother's nutritional status; 2. The structural and functional quality of the placenta; 3. The genetic makeup of the offspring; and 4. The presence of physical, chemical, or mechanical insults to mother and child during pregnancy. (McClintic, 1975).

It was previously thought that the placental membrane (it used to be called placental barrier) protected the fetus from possible damage from any of the potentially toxic drugs or substances that might be present in the mother's blood. Medical scientists now know that this was a myth. This is probably why the name was changed from barrier to membrane. The widely publicized Thalidomide disaster in 1961 demonstrated clearly that the passage of toxic substances from mother to fetus did occur and that the results could indeed be manifested in deformities that were tragic.

We are talking of very delicate mechanisms in the development of the embryo (first 2 to 8 weeks) and fetus (subsequent to 8 weeks). Medical scientists are learning more each day about the potential pathological and neurological changes that may occur in fetal development as a direct result of maternal nutritional deficiences and/or the introduction into the fetal blood of micro levels of drugs and foreign chemical substances previously thought to be harmless. Some examples of this are: Mental retardation in the offspring resulting from a maternal deficiency of iodine during the first two months of pregnancy (please recall Professor Trakhtenberg's findings regarding thyroid uptake of iodine in the presence of mercury); anticonvulsant drugs given to epileptic mothers may result in an increased incidence of cleft lip and palate, cardiac abnormalities, chromosomal aberrations, and mental deficiencies; and the maternal use of barbiturates may result in the development of hyperexcitability of brain neurons.

There is another area of concern dealing with the potential dangers associated with the drug and foreign chemicals contained in mother's milk. This area is coming under increased scientific scrutiny because, here again, there is apparently only a very limited filtering mechanism at work to preclude the introduction of these drugs and chemicals during suckling of the infant. The list of substances that may be passed to the child in this manner is truly amazing. Dr. Arena, in his 1979 book on poisons, cited approximately 150 different drugs and chemical substances excreted in human milk, covering everything from alcohol and caffeine to mercury.

The potential toxicity to the mother and her offspring associated with her total body burden of mercury cannot be ignored. Obstetricians are now cautioned to advise their patients to avoid all exposure to mercury. The scientific studies that follow clearly demonstrate the wisdom of that advice. Please pay particular attention to the study by Dr. Kuntz and his colleagues that, for the first time, clearly implicates dental fillings as contributing to the mother's total body burden of mercury:

1. Morphological (forms and structure), behavioral, and physiological (normal functioning) studies show methylmercury as having an injurious effect on the fetal nervous system even at levels which are considered not to be toxic in adults. (Reuhl and Chang, 1979; Clarkson et al, 1981; and Marsh, et al, 1980).

2. The concentration of methyl mercury in fetal blood is about 20% higher than in the mother. (Tejning, 1968).

3. The following is an abstract of the paper published by Dr. Kuntz and his co-workers in 1982. I personally consider it to be a landmark study worthy of the closest scrutiny by all health care providers, regardless of specialty. "Fifty-seven prenatal patients with no known exposure to the element mercury, or any of

its compounds, were observed for change in whole blood total mercury concentration from the initial prenatal clinic examination through delivery and postpartum hospitalization. On hospital admission for labor and delivery, whole blood total mercury averaged 1.15 parts per billion, compared to 0.79 parts per billion from the first prenatal clinic visit; these levels represent a 46% increase and significant difference in maternal concentration of a substance previously recognized for its peculiar ease at crossing the placental barrier. Previous stillbirths, as well as history of birth defects, exhibited significant positive correlation with background mercury levels. Search of the literature of the last 5 years revealed no other report of cohort heavy metal surveillance throughout pregnancy. (Kuntz, W. D.; Pitkin, R. M.; Bostrom, A. W.; and Hughes, M. S. Published in the American Journal of Obstetrics and Gynecology, Vol 143, issue 4, pages 440–443. 1982).

Dr. Kuntz concluded their study with the following statement: "Among obstetric-related historical factors, a significant association was found between previous stillbirths and mercury levels in both maternal and cord blood. Previous malformed infants significantly correlated with prenatal background mercury levels. Except for smoking early in pregnancy, none of the historical data reflecting possible mercury exposure correlated significantly with blood levels, although patients with large numbers of dental fillings exhibited a tendency to higher maternal blood mercury levels."

What is urgently needed now is for the major medical agencies and institutions to confirm and expand these findings presented by Dr. Kuntz and his associates. It also reinforces a point I made earlier regarding the necessity of considering the presence or non-presence of dental amalgam fillings if findings and conclusions derived from medical and scientific studies of humans are to be considered accurate and credible.

4. Symptoms of congenital Minamata (methylmercury) Disease included intelligence disturbances, primitive reflexes, disturbances of body growth, speech difficulties, limb deformity, hyperkinesia (hyperactivity resulting from brain damage or psychoses) and pyramidal symptoms (skilled movements, especially those of speech and those involving the hands and fingers). Mi-

crocephaly (abnormally small head/mental retardation) was present in approximately 60% of cases. The outcome was deformed, mentally retarded children and a mortality rate of approximately 7%. (Tedeschi, 1982)

5. Thirty-two infants prenatally (prior to birth) exposed to methylmercury and their mothers were studied and evaluated over a 5 year period after the Iraqi methylmercury epidemic. Although the mothers' symptoms usually improved, the damage to the fetal and infant nervous system appeared to be permanent: 1. The infants exhibited clinical manifestations of various degrees of damage to their central nervous system. 2. Ten of the 32 infants had cerebral palsy. 3. Nine of the 32 died within three years. This mortality rate of 28% compared to a 6% mortality rate in the control group (no prenatal exposure to mercury). 4. Twelve of the surviving 23 had delayed mental development; 18 showed delayed speech development; 16 showed delayed motor development; 6 had an abnormally small head circumference; and 21 exhibited hyperreflexia (exaggeration of reflexes). (Amin-Zaki and Clarkson, et al, 1979).

There are dozens of other studies that I could cite, but they all essentially confirm the findings reflected in the studies I have used. They all confirm the potential hazards of mercury exposure during pregnancy. The medical profession recognizes this fact also. Obstetricians are cautioned to advise their patients to avoid all exposure to mercury. In light of the implication of dental amalgam as a source of mercury, it would seem reasonable to also expect the medical profession to advise couples contemplating having a child about this aspect of exposure. Dental amalgam fillings should not be placed or replaced after conception because of the possibility of temporarily increasing the total body burden of mercury.

VIII.
FANTASY LAND
OR REAL PSYCHIATRIC AND BEHAVIORAL
MANIFESTATIONS?

It is apparent from the body of literature already mentioned in this book that the brain, with its component central nervous and endocrine systems, has a serious problem coping with the fact that mercury "likes" it so well.

It's like the story about the distant relative who, though uninvited, stops by to "free load" for a week-end and likes it so much that he decides to hang around until someone throws him out. Unfortunately, you only have an efficiency apartment and no matter how much you protest, your relative moves in and makes himself at home.

No matter how hard you try to ignore him and follow your normal way of life, this unwanted visitor is always under foot, getting in your way, and disrupting your regular routine. In fact, you even find him wearing your things and disguising himself to look like you. You get so frustrated you don't know what to do. What's even worse, he now looks so much like you that even some of your long time associates who look to you for advice and guidance, can't tell you apart. They even invite him into their homes to visit. However, they soon become as confused as you, because they can't figure out why you're acting so different. They can't understand why you keep playing practical jokes and tricking them into doing things they never did before.

After feeling frustrated, you become depressed. Nobody seems to understand or even want to believe in you anymore because you are so erratic. In final desperation, you decide you have to seek outside help, and go to your longtime doctor friend and tell him all you need is somebody to help you throw this unwanted visitor out, because you seem powerless to do it by yourself. He can't help, but he has a colleague that might be able to. He sets up a consultation for you with his colleague the psychiatrist, and you pour out your tale, but as intelligent and learned as he is, he doesn't seem to believe you. But, don't blame yourself, it's really his fault because nobody ever told him that the possibility even remotely existed that "unwanted visitors" could ever do this to you or anyone else.

IS THE STORY FACT OR FANTASY? Let's look at some of the facts and you judge for yourself:

1. Symptoms of methylmercury poisoning in man include psychic and behavioral disturbances. (Snyder, 1972; Kojima and Fujita, 1973; Gerstner and Huff, 1977).

2. Sixty-three persons poisoned during the 1971 Iraqi epi-

demic of methylmercury poisoning were examined. Some of the findings were: Headache occurred in 53% of the cases; 51% had sleep disturbances; 45% experienced dizziness; 42% were irritable; 12% suffered from emotional instability; and 6% were diagnosed as having mania and depression. (Damuji et al, 1976).

3. Behavioral abnormalities may occur at mercury levels below those causing clearly identifiable morphological (forms and structures) alterations and may be among the most sensitive indicators of methylmercury induced neurotoxicity (exerting a destructive or poisonous effect upon nerve tissue). (Hughes et al, 1976; Spyker, et al, 1972).

4. In another evaluation study of patients hospitalized during the second epidemic of methylmercury poisoning in Iraq that occurred in early 1972, there appeared to be a significant number suffering from depression. Of the 43 patients in the study, thirty-two (74.4%) were consistently depressed. Clinically depressive symptoms were mild to moderate in degree, consisting mainly of a feeling of depression, lack of interest, deficient concentration, and a wish to be left alone. Mercury binding compounds did not seem to have a significant effect in enhancing recovery from the depressive state. (Maghazaji, 1974).

5. Nine medical laboratory technicians who had been exposed to mercury vapor and dust were investigated. Some of the women were complaining of symptoms which were thought to be neurotic by their physicians until an investigation of three cardiac laboratories revealed significant levels of mercury in the atmosphere. The most common symptoms displayed by the technicians were: irritability, shyness, fatigue, headaches, nightmares, anxiety, tension, depression and forgetfulness. (Ross and Sholiton, 1983).

6. Metallic mercury demonstrates the importance of quantitative measures of motor function in assessing subclinical impairment (lack of positive identifiable symptoms) as well as the lack of sound psychophysiological (having bodily symptoms of an emotional origin) data about the total syndrome of mercury poisoning. Now that exposures in dental offices and laboratories are coming under increased scrutiny, psychologists might be asked what measures of psychophysiological function might help detect subclinical toxicity. Such measures could help to

identify some sources of the psychological complaints accompanying mercury intoxication. We do not have tests to recognize effects on the nervous system. There are virtually no useful tests for preclinical stages and diseases of specific organ systems such as the central nervous system. (Weiss, 1983).

Acceptance of the hypothesis that mercury in micro doses may be involved in the manifestation of psychoses is extremely difficult for the physicians who specialize in this area of medicine. It is too controversial and contrary to the accepted doctrines upon which most diagnoses are based, unless of course there has been an obvious and identifiable source of exposure to mercury. The analogy might be compared to Einstein's theory of relativity. When first expressed, it was beyond the comprehension of most other prominent physicists who maintained it wouldn't work and couldn't be proved. History, of course, proved how right Einstein was. That's where we are with micromercurialism and the art of psychiatry. All that is needed now is the "openmindedness and events" to prove or disprove the hypothesis.

REFERENCES

SECTION I

1. Steinwell, O., Transport Mechanisms in Certain Blood-Brain Barrier Phenomena—A Hypothesis. Acta Psychiatr Neurol Scand, Supplement 150, Vol 36, pages 314–318, 1961.
2. Steinwell O., and Klatzo, I., Selective Vulnerability of The Blood-Brain Barrier in Chemically Induced Lesions. Journal of Neuropathology and Experimental Neurology, Vol 25, pages 542–559, 1966.
3. Berlin, M., and Ullberg, S., Accumulation and Retentions of Mercury in The Mouse. 1. An Autoradiographic Study After A Single Intravenous Injection of Mercuric Chloride. Archives of Environmental Health (Chicago), Vol 6, pages 589–601, May 1963.
4. Broman T., and Steinwall O., Blood-Brain Barrier In: Pathology of the Nervous System. (J. Minckler Editor), Vol 1, Chapter 33. Blakeston. New York, 1967.
5. Chang L. W., and Hartman H. A., Blood-Brain Barrier Dysfunction in Experimental Mercury Intoxication. Acta Neuropathology, Vol 21, pages 179–184, 1972.

6. Ware R. A., Chang L. W., and Burkholder P. M., An Ultrastructural Study on the Blood-Brain Barrier Dysfunction Following Mercury Intoxication. Acta Neuropathology (Berlin), Vol 30, pages 211–224, 1974.

7. Yoshino Y., Mozai T., and Nakao K., Journal of Neurochemistry, Vol 13, pages 1223–1230, 1966.

8. Steinwall O., Brain Uptake of Se75-Selenomethionine After Damage to Blood-Brain Barrier by Mercuric Ions. Acta Neurologica Scandinavica, Vol 45, pages 362–368, 1969.

9. Steinwall O., and Snyder H., Brain Uptake of C^{14}—Cyclo-Leucine After Damage To Blood-Brain Barrier by Mercuric Ions. Acta Neurologica Scandinavica, Vol 45, pages 369–375, 1969.

10. Cavanagh J. B., and Chen F.C.K., Amino Acid Incorporation in Protein During the "Silent Phase" Before Organ-Mercury and P-Bromophenylacetylurea Neuropathy in the Rat. Acta Neuropathology (Berlin), Vol 19, pages 216–224, 1971.

11. Chang, L. W., Neurotoxic Effects of Mercury—A Review. Environmental Research, Vol 14, pages 329–373, 1977.

12. Schaumberger H. H., and Spencer P.S., Clinical and Experimental Studies of Distal Axonopathy—A Frequent Form of Brain and Nerve Damage Produced by Environmental Chemical Hazards. Annals of the New York Academy of Science, Vol 329, pages 14–29, 1979.

13. Gallagher P. J., and Lee R. L., The Role of Biotransformation in Organic Mercury Neurotoxicity. Toxicology, Vol 15, pages 129–134, 1980.

14. Bull R. J., and Lutkenhoff S. D., Changes in Metabolic Reponses of Brain Tissue to Stimulation, In Vitro, Produced By In Vivo Administration of Methylmercury. Neuropharmacology, Vol 14, pages 351–359, 1975.

15. Hay W. J., Richards A. G., McMenemey W. H., and Cumings J. N., Organic Mercurial Encephalopathy. Journal of Neurology and Neurosurgical Psychiatry, Vol 26, pages 199–202, June 1963.

16. Chang L. W., Mercury In: Experimental and Clinical Neurotoxicology. Williams and Wilkins, Baltimore, 1980.

17. Katsuki, et al., On the Disease of Central Nervous System in Minamata District With Unknown Etology With Special References To Clinical Observations. Kumamoto Igakki Zasshi (Suppl 23), Vol 31, pages 110–121, 1957.

18. Okinaka S., et al., Encephalomyalopathy Due To An Organic Mercury Compound. Neurology, Vol 4, pages 68–76, 1964.

19. Brown, et al., Medical Service Journal of Canada, Vol 23, page 1089, 1967.

20. Gerstner H. B., and Huff J. E., Clinical Toxicology of Mercury. Journal of Toxicology and Environmental Health, Vol 2, Issue 3, pages 491–526, 1977.

21. Rabenstein D. L., The Chemistry of Methylmercury Toxicology. Journal of Chemical Education, Vol 55, Issue 5, pages 292–296, 1978.

22. Clarkson, T. W., Biochemical Aspects of Mercury Poisoning. Journal of Occupational Medicine, Vol 10, pages 351–355, July 1968.

23. Rothstein A., Mercaptans, The Biological Targets for Mercurials In: Mercury, Mercurials and Mercaptans. Miller M. W., and Clarkson T. W. Editors, Charles C. Thomas, Springfield, Illinois, 1971.

24. Hunter, et al., Poisoning by Methylmercury Compounds. Quarterly Journal of Medicine, Vol 33, pages 193–206, 1940.

25. Garman R. H., Weiss B., and Evans H. L., Alkylmercurial Encephalopathy in The Monkey (Saimiri Scieureus and Macaca Arctoides) A Histopathologic and Autoradiographic Study. Acta Neuropathology (Berlin), Vol 32, Issuel, pages 61–74, 1975.

26. Bakir, et al., Clinical and Epidemiological Aspects of Methylmercury Poisoning. Postgraduate Medical Journal, Vol 56, pages 1–10, 1980.

27. Amin-Zaki, et al., Methylmercury Poisoning in Iraqi Children. Clinical Observations over 2 Years. British Medical Journal, Vol 1, Page 613, 1978.

28. Komulainen H., and Tuomisto J., Effect of Heavy Metals On Dopamine, Noradrenaline And Serotonin Uptake and Release In Rat Brain Synaptosomes. Acta Pharmacology and Toxicology, Vol 48, pages 199–204, 1981.

29. Ohlson C.-G., and Hogstedt C., Parkinsons Disease and Occupational Exposure to Organic Solvents, Agricultural Chemicals and Mercury—A Case Referent Study. Scandinavian Journal of Work Environment Health, Vol 7, Issue 4, pages 252–256, 1981.

SECTION II

1. Friberg L., Studies on The Metabolism of Mercuric Chloride and Methylmercury Dicyandiamide. Archives of Industrial Health, Vol 20, page 42, 1959.

2. Rodin A. E., And Crawson C. N., Mercury Nephrotoxicity in Rats: I Factors Influencing Localization of Tubular lesions. American Journal of Pathology, Vol 41, pages 297–313, 1962.

3. Joselow M. M., Goldwater L. T., and Weinberg S. B., Absorption and Excretion of Mercury in Man. Mercury Content of "Normal" Human Tissues. Archives of Environmental Health, Vol 15, Page 64, 1967.

4. Selye H., Mercury Poisoning: Prevention by Spironolcatone. Science, Vol 169, pages 775–776, 1970.

5. Wisniewska, et al., Binding of Mercury in Rat Kidney by Metallothionein. Toxicology and Applied Pharmacology, Vol 16, pages 754–763, 1970.

6. Nicholson J. K., et al., Cadmium and Mercury Nephrotoxicity. Nature, Vol 304, pages 633–635, 1983.

7. Friberg, et al., Kidney Injury After Chronic Exposure to Inorganic Mercury. Archives of Industrial Hygiene and Occupational Medicine, Vol 8, pages 149–153, 1953.

8. Kazantzis G., et al., Albuminuria And The Nephrotic Syndrome Fol-

lowing Exposure to Mercury And Its Compounds. Quarterly Journal of Medicine, Vol 31, pages 403–418, 1962.

9. OSHA Job Health Hazard Series: Mercury. OSHA 2234, August 1975.

SECTION III

1. Abraham J. E., Svare C. W., and Frank C. W., The Effect of Dental Amalgam Restorations on Blood Mercury Levels. Journal of Dental Research, Vol 63, Issue 1, pages 71–73, January 1984.

2. Kuntz W. D., et al., Maternal and Cord Blood Background Mercury Levels: A Longitudinal Surveillance. American Journal of Obstetrics and Gynecology, Vol 143, Issue 4, pages 440–443, 1982.

3. Joselow M. M., et al., Mercurialism: Environmental and Occupational Aspects. Annals of Internal Medicine, Vol 76, pages 119–130, 1972.

4. Mantyla D. G., and Wright O. D., Mercury Toxicity in The Dental Office: A Neglected Problem. Journal American Dental Association, Vol 92, pages 1189–1194, 1976.

5. Trakhtenberg I. M., et al. In: Problems of Geohygiene. Baku, page 47, 1968. Cited in Trakhtenberg Chronic Effect of Mercury on Organisms. USDHEW, PHS, NIH, DHEW Publication No. (NIH) 74–473, USGPO Washington D.C., 1974.

6. Oka M., et al., Effect of Mercuric Chloride on The Rat Mesenteric Vascular Bed: Relevance to The Mechanism of Mercury Toxicity. Toxicology and Applied Pharmacology, Vol 51, pages 427–438, 1979.

7. Chang L. W., Neurotoxic Effects of Mercury—A Review. Environmental Research, Vol 14, pages 329–373, 1977.

8. Gerstner H. B., and Huff J. E., Clinical Toxicology of Mercury. Journal of Toxicology and Environmental Health, Vol 2, Issue 3, pages 491–526, 1977.

9. Orlowski J. P., and Mercer R. D., Urine Mercury Levels in Kawasaki Disease. Pediatrics, Vol 66, Issue 4, pages 633–636, 1980.

10. Adler R., et al., Metallic Mercury Vapor Poisoning Simulating Mucocutaneous Lymph Node Syndrome. Journal of Pediatrics, Vol 101, Issue 6, pages 967–968, 1982.

11. Gregg M.B., (Editor). Kawasaki Syndrome—United States. Morbidity and Mortality Weekly Report, Vol 32, Issue 7, pages 98–100, 1983.

12. Gregg M. B., (Editor). Kawasaki Disease—New York. Morbidity and Mortality Weekly Report, Vol 29, pages 61–63, 1980.

13. Dahhan S. S., and Orfaly H., Electrocardiographic Changes in Mercury Poisoning. American Journal of Cardiology, Vol 14, pages 178–183, 1964.

14. Carmignani M., et al., Mechanisms in Cardiovascular Regulation Following Chronic Exposure of Male Rats to Inorganic Mercury. Toxicology and Applied Pharmacology, Vol 69, Issue 3, pages 442–450, 1983.

15. Cheek D. B., et al., The Effect of Mercurous Chloride (Calomel) and

Epinephrine (Sympathetic Stimulation) on Rats. The Importance of the Findings to Mechanisms in Infantile Acrodynia. Pediatrics, Vol 23, page 302, 1959.

16. Axelrod J., and Tomschick R., Enzymatic O-Methylation of Epinephrine and Other Catechols. Journal of Biological Chemistry, Vol 233, pages 702–705, 1958.

SECTION IV

1. Williams R. H., (Editor). Textbook of Endocrinology, 6th Edition, 1981. W. B. Saunders Co., Philadelphia.

2. Suzuki T., et al., Affinity of Mercury to the Thyroid. Industrial Health, Vol 4, pages 69–75, 1966.

3. Kosta L., et al., Correlation Between Selenium and Mercury in Man Following Exposure to Inorganic Mercury. Nature (London), Vol 254, pages 238–239, 1975.

4. Goldman M., and Blackburn P., The Effect of Mercuric Chloride on Thyroid Function in the Rat. Toxicology and Applied Pharmacology, Vol 48, pages 49–55, 1979.

5. Trahktenberg I. M., (See No. 5, Section III)

6. Burton B. V., and Meikle A. W., Acute and Chronic Methyl Mercury Poisoning Impairs Rat Adrenal and Testicular Function. Journal of Toxicology and Environmental Health, Vol 6, pages 597–606, 1980.

7. Khera K. S., Reproductive Capability of Male Rats and Mice Treated With Methyl Mercury. Toxicology and Applied Pharmacology, Vol 24, pages 166–177, 1973.

8. Stoewsand, et al., Eggshell Thinning in Japanese Quail Fed Mercuric Chloride. Science, Vol 173, pages 1030–1031, 1971.

9. Lee I. P., and Dixon R. L., Effects of Mercury on Spermatogenesis Studied by Velocity Sedimentation Cell Separation and Serial Mating. Journal of Pharmacology and Experimental Therapeutics, Vol 194, pages 171–181, 1975.

10. Thaxton J. P., and Parkhurst C. P., Abnormal Mating Behavior and Reproductive Dysfunction Caused by Mercury in Japanese Quail. Proceedings Society of Experimental Biology and Medicine, Vol 144, pages 252–255, 1973.

11. Diamond S. S., and Sleight S. D., Acute and Sub-Chronic Methylmercury Toxicosis in the Rat. Toxicology and Applied Pharmacology, Vol 23, pages 197–207, 1972.

12. Kojima K., and Fujita M., Summary of Recent Studies in Japan on Methylmercury Poisoning. Toxicology, Vol 1, pages 43–62, 1973.

13. Alomar A., et al., Addison's Disease and Contact Dermatitis from Mercury in Soap. Contact Dermatitis, Vol 9, Issue 1, page 76, 1983.

SECTION V

1. Stites D. P., Stobo J. D., Fundenberg H. H., and Wells J. V., Basic and Clinical Immunology, 4th Edition, 1982. Lange Medical Publications, Los Altos, CA.

2. Williams R. H., (See No. 1, Section IV)

3. McClintic J. R., Physiology of The Human Body. John Wiley & Sons, Inc., N.Y., 1975.

4. Homberger F., Hayes J. A., and Pelikan E. W., (Editors). A Guide to General Toxicology. Karger AG, Basel, Switzerland, 1983.

5. Verschaeve L., et al., Genetic Damage Induced by Occupational Low Mercury Exposure. Environmental Research, Vol 12, pages 306–316, 1976.

6. Popescu H. I., et al., Chromosome Aberration Induced by Occupational Exposure to Mercury. Archives of Environmental Health, Vol 34, Issue 6, pages 461–463, 1979.

7. Skerfving S., Hansson K., and Linstren J., Chromosome Breakage in Humans Exposed to Methylmercury Through Fish Consumption. Archives of Environmental Health, Vol 21, pages 133–139, 1970.

8. Skerving S., et al., Methylmercury-Induced Chromosome Damage in Man. Environmental Research, Vol 7, pages 83–98, 1974.

9. Fiskesjo G., The Effect of Two Organic Mercury Compounds on Human Leukocytes In Vitro. Hereditas, Vol 64, pages 142–146, 1970.

10. Weening J. J., Chapter 4, Mercury Induced Immune Complex Glomerulopathy: An Experimental Study. Van Dan Denergen, 1980.

11. Blakley, et al., The Effect of Methylmercury, Tetraethyl Lead and Sodium Arsenite on The Humoral Response in Mice. Toxicology and Applied Pharmacology, Vol 52, pages 245–254, 1980.

12. Koller L. D., Immunosuppression Produced by Lead, Cadmium and Mercury. American Journal of Veterinary Research, Vol 34, page 1457, 1973.

13. Koller L. D., Immunotoxicology of Heavy Metals. International Journal of Immunopharmacology, Vol 2, pages w69–279, 1980.

14. Schopf E., Schultz K. H., and Gromm M., Transformationen Und Mitosen Vun Lymphozyten In Vitro Durch Quecksilber (11)-Chlorid. Naturwissenschaften, Vol 54, page 568, 1967.

16. Caron G. A., Poutala S., and Provost T. T., Lymphocyte Transformation Induced by Inorganic and Organic Mercury. International Archives of Allergy and Applied Immunology, Vol 37, pages 76–87, 1970.

SECTION VI

1. Frykholm K. O., On Mercury From Dental Amalgam Its Toxic and Allergic Effects and Some Comments on Occupational Hygiene. Acta Odontologica Scandinavica, Vol 15, Supplement 22, pages 1–108, 1957.

2. Schafer, et al., A Textbook of Oral Pathology. W. B. Saunders Co., Philadelphia, 1974.

3. Goodman and Gillman's, The Pharmacological Basis of Therapeutics. 6th Edition, 1980. Macmillan Publishing Co., Inc. New York.

4. Bergenholtz A., Multiple Polypous Hyperplasias of the Oral Mucosa With Regression After Removal of Amalgam Fillings. Acta Odontologica Scandinavica, Vol 23, Issue 2, pages 111–131, April 1965.

5. Zander, H. A., Effect of Silicate Cement and Amalgam on the Gingiva. Journal American Dental Association, Vol 55, page 11, 1957.

6. App G. R., Effect of Silicate, Amalgam and Cast Gold on the Gingiva. Journal of Prosthetic Dentistry, Vol 11, page 522, 1961.

7. Freden H., et al., Mercury Content in Gingival Tissues Adjacent to Amalgam Fillings. Odontologica Review, Vol 25, Issue 2, pages 207–210, 1974.

8. Till T., and Maly K., Zum Nachweis Der Lyse Von Hg Aus Silber-Amalgam Von Zahnfullungen. Der Praktesche Arzt, Vol 32, page 1042, 1978.

SECTION VII

1. McClintic J. R., (See No. 3, Sect V)

2. Arena, J., Poisoning, 4th Edition, 1979. Charles C. Thomas, Springfield, Illinois.

3. Kuntz N. D., et al., Maternal and Cord Blood Background Mercury Levels: A Longitudinal Surveillance. American Journal of Obstetrics and Gynecology, Vol 143, pages 440–443, 1982.

4. Reuhl K. R., and Chang L. W., Neurotoxicology, Vol 1, pages 21–55, 1979.

5. Clarkson T. W., et al., Dose-Response Relationships for Adult Prenatal Exposures to Methylmercury. In: Measurement of Risks, G. G., and Mialle H. D., (Editors). Plenum, New York, 1981.

6. Marsh D. O., et al., Fetal Methylmercury Poisoning: Clinical and Toxicological Data on 29 Cases. Annals of Neurology, Vol 7, pages 348–453, 1980.

7. Tejning S., Mercury Levels in Blood Corpuscles and in Plasma in "Normal" Mothers and Their New-Born Children, Report 68 02 Z from Dept of Occupational Medicine, University Hospital, Lund Sweden, Lung Stencils, 1968.

8. Tedeschi L. G., The Minamata Disease. American Journal of Forensic Medicine and Pathology, Vol. 3, Issue 4, pages 335–338, 1982.

9. Amin Zaki L., et al. and Clarkson T. W., et al., Prenatal Methylmercury Poisoning. American Journal Disabled Children, Vol. 133, pages 172–177, 1979.

SECTION VIII

1. Snyder, R. D., The Involuntary Movements of Chronic Mercury Poisoning. Archives of Neurology, Vol 26, pages 379–381, 1972.

2. Kojima, K., and Fujita, M., Summary of Recent Studies in Japan on Methylmercury Poisoning. Toxicology, Vol. 1, Issue 1, pages 43–62, 1973.

3. Gerstner H. B., and Huff, J. E., Clinical Toxicology of Mercury. Journal of Toxicology and Environmental Health, Vol. 2, Issue 3, pages 491–526, 1977.

4. Damuji S. F., and The Clinical Committee on Mercury Poisoning, Intoxication Due to Alkyl-Mercury Treated Seed—1971–1972-Outbreak in Iraq Clinical Aspects, Bulletin World Health Organization, Vol. 53, (Suppl), page 65, 1976.

5. Spyker, J. M., et al., Subtle Consequences of Methyl Mercury Exposure: Behavioral Deviations in Offspring of Treated Mothers. Science, Vol. 177, pages 621–623, 1972.

6. Maghazaji, H. I., Psychiatric Aspects of Methylmercury Poisoning. Journal of Neurology, Neurosurgery and Psychiatry, Vol. 37, Issue 8, pages 954–958, 1974.

7. Ross, W. D., and Sholiton, M. C., Specificity of Psychiatric Manifestations in Relation to Neurotoxic Chemicals. Acta Psychiatry Scandinavia, Vol. 67, Suppl 303, pages 100–104, 1983.

8. Weiss, B., Behavioral Toxicology and Environmental Health Science. Opportunity and Challenge for Psychology. American Psychologist, Nov 1983, pages 1174–1187.

CHAPTER 8

MICROMERCURIALISM
AND SIGNS AND SYMPTOMS
MERCURY CAN PRODUCE

Although there are references to micro doses and micromercurialsm in several places in the book, I haven't attempted to define it previously. Micromercurialism was first described by Professor Stock in 1926 on the basis of psychological changes observed in persons chronically exposed to low concentrations of atmospheric mercury. Professor Trakhtenberg in his 1969 monograph called the micromercurialism defined by Stock an "asthenic-vegetative syndrome".

Dorland's Illustrated Medical Dictionary does not list micromercurialism or carry the asthenic-vegetative syndrome under their listing of established syndromes. However, it does define the terms: asthenic is defined as "pertaining to or characterized by asthenia." Asthenia is defined as "lack or loss of strength and energy; weakness." Of the six major categories of asthenia defined, the three considered most pertinent to our discussion are: "asthenia gravis hypophyseogenea, a pituitary dysfunction marked by emaciation, anorexia, constipation, amenorrhea, hypothermia, hypotonia, and hypoglycemia. Myalgic asthenia, a condition in which the general symptoms are a sensation of general fatigue and muscular pains. Neurocirculatory asthenia, a symptom complex characterized by the occurrence of breathlessness, giddiness, a sense of fatigue, pain in the chest in the region of the precordium, and palpitation. It occurs chiefly in soldiers in active war service, though it is seen in civilians also. Called also effort syndrome, cardiac neurosis, DaCosta's disease or syndrome, anxiety neurosis, neurasthenia, cardiasthenia, cardiac neurasthenia and cardioneurosis." Vegetative is defined as "functioning involuntarily or unconsciously, as the vegetative nervous system; (an old term for the autonomic nervous system)."

Professor Trakhtenberg states in his monograph that Professor Stock characterized micromercurialism symptoms in three groups according to their degree of intensity of the phenomenon. "First degree micromercurialism results in lowered work capacity, increased fatigue, light nervous excitability. Often in the second degree there is swelling of the nasal membranes, progressive weakening of memory, feelings of fear and loss of self-confidence, irritability, headaches. Simultaneously there may be catarrhal symptoms and upper respiratory discomfort, changes in the mucous membranes of the mouth, bleeding gums. Sometimes there are feelings of coronary insufficiency, shivering, quickening pulse, and a tendency toward diarrhea. Third degree micromercurialism is characterized by symptoms approaching those of regular mercurialism, but to a lesser degree. The basic symptoms of this stage are: headaches, general weakness, sleeplessness, decline in intellectual capacity, depression. Among other signs are tears, diarrhea, frequent urination, a feeling of pressure in the cardiac region and shivering." Please keep in mind that Professor Stock stated his findings in 1926.

Professor Trakhtenberg also cited reports by A. M. Gel'fand (1928), and A. N. L'vov (1939) that focus on the difficulty of diagnosing micromercurialism. Gel'fand found that sometimes mercury poisoning in patients was mistaken for other diseases and L'vov cited cases of micromercurialism misdiagnosed as neurasthenia, hysteria, etc. He further noted that although there were only a few cases of chronic mercury poisoning reported among mercury industry workers, qualified pathologists frequently reported the phenomenon of micromercurialism among this same class of mercury workers.

Professor Trakhtenberg concludes in his monograph that clinical micromercurialism shows characteristic symptoms of its own in addition to the classical symptoms of chronic mercury poisoning. These were attributed to disturbances in the cortical centers of the central nervous system and are manifested by functional changes in organs of the cardiovascular, urogenital, or endocrine systems. (NIOSH, Occupational Exposure to Inorganic Mercury, 1973).

Again, and as most scientists that have studied micromercurialism have concluded, further study, toxicological experimentation and additional clinical observations are needed.

SIGNS AND SYMPTOMS
ELEMENTAL MERCURY VAPOR EXPOSURE

1. **Psychological disturbances (erethism):**
   - Irritability
   - Nervousness
   - Shyness or timidity
   - Loss of memory
   - Lack of attention
   - Loss of self-confidence
   - Decline of intellect
   - Lack of self control
   - Fits of anger
   - Depression
   - Anxiety
   - Drowsiness
   - Insomnia
2. **Oral Cavity Disorders:**
   - Bleeding gums
   - Alveolar bone loss
   - Loosening of teeth
   - Excessive salivation
   - Foul breath
   - Metallic taste
   - Leukoplakia
   - Stomatitis
   - Ulceration of gingiva, palate, tongue
   - Burning sensation in mouth or throat
   - Tissue pigmentation

3. **Gastrointestinal Effects:**
   Abdominal cramps
   Gastrointestinal problems, colitis
   Diarrhea
4. **Systemic Effects:**
Cardiovascular:
   Irregular heartbeat (tachycardia, bradycardia)
   Feeble and irregular pulse
   Alterations in blood pressure
   Pain or pressure in chest
Neurologic:
   Chronic or frequent headaches
   Dizziness
   Ringing or noises in ears
   Fine tremors: hands, feet, lips, eyelids, tongue
Respiratory:
   Persistent cough
   Emphysema
   Shallow and irregular respiration
Immunological:
   Allergies
   Asthma
   Rhinitis
   Sinusitis
   Lymphadenopathy, especially cervical
Endocrine:
   Subnormal temperature
   Cold, clammy skin, especially hands and feet
   Excessive perspiration
   Muscle weakness
   Fatigue
   Anemia
   Hypoxia
   Edema
   Loss of appetite (anorexia)
   Loss of weight
   Joint pains

5. **Severe Cases:**
      Hallucinations
      Manic-depression
ORGANIC MERCURY EXPOSURE
1. **Earliest Symptoms**
      Fatigue
      Headache
      Forgetfulness
      Inability to concentrate
      Apathy
      Depression
      Outbursts of anger
      Decline of intellect
2. **Later Findings:**
      Numbness and tingling of hands, feet, lips
      Muscle weakness progressing to paralysis
      Dim or restricted vision
      Hearing difficulty
      Speech disorders
      Loss of memory
      Incoordination
      Emotional instability
      Dermatitis
      Renal damage
      General central nervous system dysfunctions
3. **Late Symptoms**
      Coma
      Death

The problem with a listing of signs and symptoms is that they can apply to so many other diseases, syndromes, or impaired health conditions. I caution everyone not to jump to conclusions. However, I also urge anyone with a mouth full of silver amalgam fillings and a collection of the signs and symptoms listed, who has repeatedly sought medical help in determining the cause, and has not received a conclusive diagnosis or treatment, to pursue the matter further.

It won't be easy. The prevailing attitude within the medical and dental communities will probably subject you to a "professorial" lecture on the ridiculousness of a question like "Doctor could the mercury in my amalgam fillings have any bearing on my condition?" Or, the question might be summarilly dismissed. Or, you may even be considered a likely candidate for psychological evaluation. Don't be deterred. You are entitled to the most serious consideration of your "question", especially if you have been under the care of a physician who has not been able to tell you what is causing your health problems. A subsequent chapter deals with what you can do to get an intelligent answer.

Many of the scientific papers investigating the mercury phenomenon have determined that some of the signs and symptoms associated with mercury exposure will ameliorate or disappear if the source of exposure is eliminated. This is possible if the cells of the impaired organs or function have not been damaged irreparably. It is accomplished simply by removing the source, and/ or administering drugs or nutrients that tend to normalize function by binding with the mercury and removing it from the body via the urine or feces.

The key phrase in the above statement and in many of the scientific studies that have been done is "irreparable cell damage". Unfortunately, we are talking about very subtle and insidious cell damage that in most instances was never even looked for, or determined, because the studies or experiments were only attempting to determine one specific fact. The experiment protocols were simply not designed to detect possible cell damage in some other organ or system of the body.

As a result, many of our leading authorities in medicine and science tend to minimize the potential toxic effects of mercury except in those instances where there has been intoxication from known exposure. The operative words in that statement are INTOXICATION and KNOWN EXPOSURE. Micromercurialism I am afraid, never enters the picture.

This could be truly unfortunate for the millions of us who may be accumulating mercury in our bodies attributable to microdoses emanating from dental amalgam. The diagnosis, at best, is difficult and will be impossible if the health care provider you are seeing doesn't believe micromercurialism exists to begin with. How can you diagnose something if you don't believe it exists? Under that situation, the diagnostician is trying to tie your symptomatology to one of the diseases and/or conditions already defined and contained in the medical literature.

REFERENCES

1. Goodman and Gillman's. The Pharmacological Basis of Therapeutics. 6th Edition, 1980. Macmillan Publishing Co., Inc., New York.

2. Dorland's Illustrated Medical Dictionary. 25th Edition, 1974. W. B. Saunders Co., Philadelphia.

3. Report of an International Committee: Maximum allowable concentrations of mercury compounds. (MAC Values). Archives of Environmental Health, Vol. 19: pages 891–905, 1969.

4. Criteria for a recommended standard: Occupational Exposure to Inorganic Mercury. U.S. Department of Health, Education, and Welfare. Public Health Service. National Institute for Occupational Safety and Health, 1973.

4. Schafer, et al. A Textbook of Oral Pathology. 1974. W. B. Saunders Co., Philadelphia.

5. Trakhtenberg, I. M., Chronic Effects of Mercury on Organisms. U.S. Department of Health, Education, and Welfare. Publication Number (NIH) 74–473, 1974.

6. Gerstner, H. B., and Huff, J. E. Clinical Toxicology of Mercury. Journal of Toxicology and Environmental Health, Vol. 2, issue 3: pages 491–526, 1977.

7. Elhassani, S. B., The Many Faces of Methylmercury Poisoning. Journal of Toxicology: Clinical Toxicology, Vol. 19 issue 8, pages 875–906, 1982–1983.

8. Chang, L. W., Mercury In: Experimental and Clinical Neurotoxicology. Williams and Wilkins, 1980.

9. Mantyla, D. G., and Wright, O. D., Mercury Toxicity in The Dental Office: A Neglected Problem. Journal American Dental Association, Vol. 92, pages 1189–1194, 1976.

CHAPTER 9

ANECDOTES

Some of the dentists practicing mercury-free dentistry have been kind enough to provide me with some anecdotes or case histories. These all involve real, live people and are not figments of my imagination, the dentists', or the patients'. All of the case histories reflect documentation contained in either the dental records or the patient health history forms of the individuals concerned. Some I have personally interviewed. No names or locations have been included.

As stated in Chapter 2, anecdotal histories are normally not acceptable to the scientific community because they cannot be presented as statistical evidence and as a general rule are subject to human bias. It is a scientific fact that with some people, just the power of suggestion can cause the body to react in a favorable response. These are the individuals who after the administration of a "placebo" respond the same as if they had been administered medication. At least temporarily anyway.

From the researcher's standpoint, using or relating anecdotal evidence can be extremely frustrating. It immediately opens the door for criticism by his peers, be they dentist, physician or scientist. Those who criticize are also prone to disregard the hypothesis being developed through use of the anecdotes. For these individuals it is impossible for them to accept any evidence that is not derived from animal studies, or blind/double blind clinical trials. Therein lies a real tragedy for humanity. Mankind would be much better served if all those quick to denigrate would instead view the hypotheses and anecdotal histories objectively. If fully documented case histories are provided, together with a rational hypothesis, a more intelligent reaction would be to see if there was some scientific basis that could be proved, or disproved, through conventional research.

There is nothing wrong with healthy skepticism. However, it is slightly bizzare that a physician or group of physicians who may have diagnosed a major medical disease in a particular individual cannot accept as the truth, any amelioration in symptoms or an actual cure that doesn't result from the administration of a prescribed drug and/or surgery. I am not implying that all physicians feel that way. There are a great number of health care providers whose only concern is "that you were helped", regardless of the protocol.

There are a couple of serious cautions or warnings for those of you who feel any of the case histories sound exactly like your own situation. Don't assume anything and don't take any precipitous action without sound medical and dental advice. Chapter 10, outlines some courses of action that you as individuals can take. Read it carefully and proceed cautiously.

CASE 1

The individual is a white male who at the time of treatment was 61 years old. He is an engineer who had been exposed to mercury containing instruments most of his working life, ie., manometers, thermometers, etc., and also frequently had elemental mercury stored in his home.

He had previously been the patient of another dentist who did not believe anything about the potential toxicity of mercury from dental amalgam. Wanting to explore the problem further, he sought out his present dentist (who practices mercury-free dentistry) to get an evaluation as to whether mercury could possibly be involved in any of his varied health problems.

On November 11, 1983 he had his first appointment with the new dentist. The examination revealed that the patient had 6 amalgam surfaces (2 upper right and 4 upper left). He also had a 4 unit nickle/porcelain bridge on the lower left and a 3 unit nickle/porcelain bridge on the lower right. A complete medical history was taken and he was then evaluated for possible mercury toxicity/hypersensitivity. His diagnosis was possible mercury intoxication and the dentist recommended removal and replacement of the amalgam fillings with a composite. It was also recommended that the nickle bridges be replaced because of their potential carcinogenicity.

The patient's health history taken at the time of the initial visit revealed the following:

First amalgam fillings installed in 1943. Suffered incident of convulsions shortly thereafter. Also developed an allergic reaction to scallops shortly after placement of the fillings.

In 1945, while overseas with the armed forces, had 21 amalgam filling surfaces installed. Developed eczema right after the dental work was completed and was hospitalized for six months during which time he almost had one of his legs amputated because of the severity of the eczema.

In 1960, a gold bridge was installed on the upper right. He was hospitalized 1–2 months later with nausea and vomiting. He was diagnosed as having an ulcer, but did not respond to treatment. His immune system was found to be depressed and he was given antibiotics by IV.

During 1980–1981, patient was hospitalized 7 times. Diagnosed as having an inflamed pancreas that should be removed. Patient refused surgery. Was also diagnosed as having some deterioration of the right kidney, gall bladder, and liver.

Patient has had: continuous ear infections for 34 years; chronic headaches that would start in the occipital region, all of his adult life; for the past 15 years joint pains especially in his wrists and knees; abdominal pains for 30 years; paresthesia in his feet the last three years; tremors in his right arm and left leg; occasional uncontrollable hiccups; occasional chest pains and constipation; occasional cardiac bradycardia and missed beats; loss of visual accommodation; farsighted in the early 1960's. Patient says he is irritable, experiences anxiety, is unable to concentrate and feels he has had a decrease in memory, has suffered a loss of libido, is more introverted (shy), and has had an erythemetous rash, with itching and burning, especially on his legs, sternum and right facial cheek.

No depression, no fits of anger or loss of self control, no nightmares, and hearing is O.K.

Patient was referred to an M.D. for a coordinated protocol on Jan 11, 1984. On Feb 6, 1984, M.D. advised dentist that patient had recovered from a bleeding ulcer and that he would administer Vitamin C by IV the morning of his first dental appointment which was then scheduled for March 7, 1984.

March 7, 1984: 6 amalgam surfaces replaced with composite. (2 upper right and 4 upper left).

March 15, 1984: Removed 4 unit nickle/porcelain bridge from lower left. There were three amalgam surfaces under the bridge which were then replaced with composite.

March 22, 1984: Removed 3 unit nickle/porcelain bridge from lower right.

March 29, 1984: Delivered new porcelain fused to gold 4 unit bridge to lower left. Patient stated he is "feeling much better every week. Back pain is now totally gone".

April 5, 1984: Delivered new 3 unit porcelain fused to gold bridge to lower right. Patient stated "I am feeling great now". The patient also presented the dentist with a list of his symptoms and their chronology since he had started treatment. Changes in patient symptomatology started to occur on March 11, 1984: sneezing and headaches decreased but back pain and eczema increased. By March 27: back pain, neck stiffness, sneezing, coughing, eczema had all noticibly decreased. Headaches, dry throat and tooth aches had all ceased. By April 5, 1984: all symptoms had ceased with the exception of the eczema and earaches which had both decreased from moderate to light.

June 26, 1984: In a follow-up conversation with me the patient stated that the eczema and earaches had cleared entirely.

CASE 2

This 45 year-old Caucasian female was first seen by the dentist on April 8, 1983. She had requested the appointment after reading a newspaper article concerning the potential toxicity of dental amalgam. The dental examination included full mouth x-rays, evaluation of electrogalvanic potentials and a full consultation. The patient had a total of 30 amalgam surfaces in 11 teeth. Her health history and consultation revealed the following facts:

1980: Went to see her physician because of a numb feeling in her right nasal ala. Subsequent tests revealed liver abnormalities and neuritis. Patient was hospitalized for neurological evaluation, and other tests. The neurologist stated "right side not as good as left side. There was paresthesia on the entire right side of body". Bone scan, liver, spleen, skull, and barium enema were all normal. Resultant diagnosis was possibly "nerves".

Patient went to a chiropractor for an adjustment, who stated that she was slightly out of alignment, especially the atlas and occipitus. However, after adjustment, her body would not remain in alignment.

Patient went to visit another M.D. This physician stated he thought her problems might be related to mercury toxicity from her dental fillings because her throat was always red and burning (without any infection). Her nose was always stuffed; there was a pain in her right eye; a horrible taste in her mouth; joint pains in her right shoulder, elbow, knee and ankle. Patient also had consulted with a dermatologist concerning a skin rash which she frequently had all over her body. The dermatologist was unable to determine any cause for the rash.

The dental examination also revealed swollen lymph nodes under the right side of jaw and a click in the right TMJ. Dental diagnosis was possible mercury intoxication, with a recommendation that all dental amalgams be replaced with composites. The first appointment was scheduled for April 25, 1983.

4/25/83: Amalgams removed from 3 teeth on lower right (8 surfaces) and replaced with composite.

5/2/83: Patient stated "I can breathe a little better on my right side now. My hands and right side of my face are not as swollen. I started to notice improvement within hours of the initial amalgam replacement done on 4/25/83". Amalgams were removed from 3 teeth on the upper right (9 surfaces) and replaced with composites.

5/9/83: Patient's right nostril is completely clear now and

left nostril is opening slightly. Patient has noticed improvements 6 to 7 hours after removal of amalgams each time. Patient also has had green bowel movements after each session. Amalgams removed in 3 teeth (4 surfaces on lower left and 2 surfaces on upper right) and replaced with composites.

5/16/83: Remaining amalgams in 2 teeth (6 surfaces upper left) removed and replaced with composites. A total of 30 amalgam surfaces had been removed and replaced during the treatment plan.

2/17/84: Patient reported that she was doing great. There were no more breathing problems or swelling. Stated her physician wanted to know what she had done to improve so.

6/27/84: In a follow-up conversation with me, the patient stated that she was "much better all the way around". No more headaches, no metallic taste in her mouth, no more breathing problems or sore throat, and no more pressure build up behind her right eye.

CASE 3

Patient is a 48 year-old Caucasian female who was referred to this office by another dentist for determination of electrogalvanic potentials. The other dentist had administered a mercury patch test on August 26, 1983, which was positive but he did not want to remove the patient's amalgam fillings. On September 20, 1983, her first visit to the new dentist, there was still a red raised wheal at the site of the patch test area. The patient was examined and a health history taken that revealed the following information:

Patient had been diagnosed as having Lupus Erythemetosis two years previously. She had just gotten over a bad staph infection in her left eye for which she had received treatment at a medical clinic. Since then she had become allergic to codeine and sulfa drugs. Her previous dentist had advised her that she was also allergic to nickel. (Examination revealed a nickel-based porcelain to metal crown on the lower left 1st bicuspid).

Patient has had gastro-intestinal problems for the past 7–8 years; skin reactions for 15 years; far sightedness the last 6–7 years. No arthritis, no heart problems, no paresthesia, no tinnitus, and no headaches. Patient stated her skin rash had become worse 2 years ago, especially on neck, chest, stomach, and thighs.

Patient had 38 amalgam surfaces on 12 teeth. Dental diagnosis was possible mercury intoxication with a recommendation that all amalgam fillings be replaced with composites. First appointment was scheduled for November 2, 1983.

11/2/83: Area of mercury patch test still red and had a raised wheal. Amalgam fillings were removed from upper left 2nd molar (4 surfaces) and replaced with composite.

11/9/83: Patient reported she felt headachy after last appointment and the following day. Also had pain in lower right back the day following last appointment. Amalgam fillings were removed from 3 teeth on upper left (10 surfaces) and replaced with composites.

11/15/83: Amalgam fillings were removed from 3 teeth on lower left (9 surfaces) and replaced with composites.

11/30/83: Patient stated she has had intermittent dull headaches since last appointment but that they were beginning to ease. She also had a Lupus rash breakout on the medial and dorsal left ankle and medial left flank. Amalgam fillings removed from lower right (10 surfaces) and replaced with composites. Patient was feeling weak and nauseous after procedure. Blood pressure was 132/80.

12/7/83: Amalgam fillings removed on upper and lower right (9 surfaces) and replaced with composites.

1/11/84: Patient's Lupus Erythemous symptoms much improved. No more skin rashes. Eyesight seems better and eyes are less sensitive and not red. Removed crown on lower left 1st bicuspid and placed temporary composite full crown.

1/17/84: Patient reported eyes were red and irritated for 3 days after crown was removed. Physical condition much improved. No more skin rashes. Mouth less and less sensitive every day.

6/27/84: I called the patient to confirm the information contained in the dental records. The patient stated that her diagnosed Lupus condition had manifested itself primarily as skin rashes and that since replacement of her amalgam fillings she had been symptom free. She also stated that her eyes, which had always been bloodshot and for which she continually had to use eye drops, were no longer red. More importantly she said that the pressure build-up behind her eyes had disappeared.

CASE 4

Patient is a 37 year-old Caucasian male who was first seen on April 2, 1983. In October 1966, while on military service, patient had 4 small pit amalgam fillings placed. These were his first and only fillings. Patient's health history revealed the following:

October 1967: Hospitalized for severe malaise, lack of muscular control, could not walk. Base military hospital could not determine cause. Was sent to Chelsea Navy Hospital in Boston for further evaluation. A specific diagnosis could not be made but Multiple Sclerosis was suspected. Patient was discharged from military service. During the 1966–1967 period patient began wearing glasses, to correct for a myopic (near sighted) condition.

August 11, 1982: Hospitalized as a result of a heart attack. Suffered two more heart attacks during the next two weeks while still in the hospital. One week after 1st heart attack patient had kidney failure and was on dialysis for 72 days (as a result of all his health problems, he also lost his job). Patient had suffered pain in all major joints of body for 1 year prior to heart attack which became worse after his heart attacks. Also had chronic headaches for 4 months prior to heart attacks and had noticed diminished hearing during the year prior to his initial heart attack. Patient had been experiencing light-headedness and dizziness for 3–4 years prior to heart attacks and had also noticed a loss of short term memory during this same period.

While hospitalized for his heart attack, patient was diagnosed as being diabetic, although he had no previous history of diabetes. Had pancreatitis 1 month after heart attack, and also had his spleen removed at that time. Attending physician stated that patient's liver looked bad (patient states he was virtually a teatotaller and had no previous history of liver problems).

Patient had brought with him to his first appointment xrays from previous dentist. An electrogalvanic evaluation was done, and after consultation with patient, treatment plan for removal and replacement of amalgams was agreed to. At this time the patient's vital signs were: pulse 66, temperature 98.0, blood pressure, left arm 120/80, right arm 120/80. First appointment scheduled for April 13, 1983.

April 13, 1983: Vital signs prior to performing any dental work: pulse 78, temperature 97, blood pressure 118/80. Two small pit amalgam fillings on the upper right were removed and replaced with composite fillings. Vital signs 15 minutes after completion of dental work: pulse 72, temperature 98.6, blood pressure 120/84.

April 15, 1983: 2nd appointment. Patient stated his joint pains had totally cleared up for the first time since leaving the Navy and that he felt "good and stronger". Vital signs prior to dental work: pulse 68, temperature 98.0, blood pressure 120/74. Two small pit amalgam fillings on the upper left and lower right were removed and replaced with composite fillings. Vital signs 15 minutes after completion of dental work: pulse 68, temperature 98.0, blood pressure 120/80.

5/23/83: Patient called to say he was "doing great", no joint pains and feels better all around. Worked in the yard the first time in 7 years.

Patient has subsequently regained employment.

6/27/84: In a conversation with the patient he stated that replacement of his amalgam fillings had helped clear all of the problems he had previously reported.

CASE 5

Patient is a 47 year-old Caucasian female who called for the appointment after hearing a local radio talk show discussing the possibility of mercury toxicity from dental amalgam fillings.

Patient's health history revealed the following:

Bilateral mastectomy with mammoplasty due to fibrocystic nonmalignant lumps were performed in 1976. Three months later a hysterectomy was done to stop excessive bleeding.

Patient suffers with insomnia and cannot sleep more than one hour at a time; gets frequent headaches which start at back of neck; fatigues easily; has coordination difficulties; vision difficulties at times and chronic eye inflammation; has edema and is constantly thirsty; chest pains; abdominal pain; generalized arthritic condition not relieved by aspirin; is depressed with occasional thoughts of suicide; has throat constrictions. Patient also stated she gets excrutiating pain throughout body which triggers spasms in her jaw, feels like she will convulse. The pain and jaw spasms started immediately after new braces were put on by her orthodontist.

Patient was given a mercury patch test. Vital signs prior to patch test were: pulse 78, temperature 99.0, blood pressure 102/70. One hour after patch was applied vital signs were: pulse 70, temperature 90, blood pressure 115/72. Patient got tingly, prickly sensation in mouth. Patch was removed and test terminated because of reactions. Diagnosis was a positive reaction to the mercury patch test.

Patient had 38 amalgam surfaces in 16 teeth. A treatment plan was discussed and agreed to and the first appoinment was scheduled for July 1, 1983.

7/1/83: Amalgams removed from three teeth on lower left (8 surfaces) and replaced with composite fillings.

7/4/83: Patient was called to see how she was doing. Patient stated "best I've felt in 10 years, slept four hours straight. Cleaned the house and still had energy".

7/5/83: Patient called at 4:15 P.M. and stated she was having symptoms of diarrhea, a sensation of bladder or kidney infection starting, and was passing blood in urine. She was told to contact her physician immediately and that her appointment for 7/6/83 would be cancelled.

7/6/83: Patient called at 8:15 A.M. and stated she was doing 100% better. Her appointment was rescheduled for 7/9/83.

7/9/83: Amalgams removed from four teeth on lower right (11 surfaces) and replaced with composite fillings.

7/13/83: Dentist consulted with the orthodontist and both agreed patient would be better off with braces removed. Amalgams removed from four teeth upper left (6 surfaces) and replaced with composite fillings.

7/16/83: Remaining amalgams removed from five teeth on upper right (13 surfaces) and replaced with composite fillings.

6/27/83: I called patient to confirm information reflected on the dental records. During the course of the conversation patient brought out the fact that she had also been diagnosed as having Multiple Sclerosis and that this condition was now cleared up. She attributed the resolution of the MS to the removal and replacement of the amalgam fillings and to subsequent treatment received from a holistic physician. During the latter treatment an allergy to wheat was diagnosed and she has carefully avoided wheat to the best of her ability.

CASE 6

he patient is a 58 year-old Oriental female who was first seen on June 24, 1983. Consultation and patient health history revealed the following information:

Patient stated she was diagnosed as having rheumatoid arthritis in 1957 approximately two years after having all her amalgam fillings removed and replaced with new amalgam fillings. Her dentist in Maryland advised her to have this done because her old fillings were deteriorating and there was decay under some of the fillings. Patient moved to Florida in 1958 and had taken aspirin for her arthritis condition for over 20 years. Patient had undergone gold treatments for her arthritis but had developed a rash. She had also had DMSO treatments which seemed to help her arthritis. Patient has a raw burning feeling in mouth and throat and has suffered some loss of hearing. Patient had knot on back of right hand and stated she had similar knots all over her body. Also stated she was very allergic to poison ivy.

Patient was given a mercury patch test. Vital signs prior to test were: pulse 88, temperature 98.6, blood pressure 104/66. Vital signs one hour after patch was applied: pulse 90, temperature 99, blood pressure 116/78. Patch test was terminated with a diagnosis of positive reaction to mercury.

Patient had 26 amalgam surfaces in 14 teeth. Patient also had one gold inlay. A treatment plan was discussed and agreed to with the first appointment scheduled for July 13, 1983.

7/13/83: Amalgams removed from three teeth on lower left (7 surfaces) and replaced with composite fillings. Removed gold inlay from lower left 1st bicuspid. There was an amalgam filling under the gold and the tooth had necrotic (dead) pulp. Placed temporary crown and recommended that root canal therapy be performed.

7/20/83: Amalgams removed from two teeth on lower right (7 surfaces) and replaced with composite fillings.

8/5/83: Amalgams removed from two teeth on upper right (4 surfaces) and replaced with composite fillings.

8/17/83: Amalgams removed from four teeth on upper left (8 surfaces) and replaced with composite fillings.

10/3/83: Patient called and stated she is getting better very slowly. Joints are not quite as sore.

11/4/83: Patient called and stated she is gradually getting better.

11/9/83: Impression taken for replacement crown.

11/29/83: Patient stated swelling in hands and joints has gone down considerably and that she has increased gripping strength in both hands. Delivered porcelain fused to gold full crown with cast gold core.

6/27/84: I called the patient to see what her physical condition was 7 months after treatment had been completed. The patient stated that her arthritis condition had ameliorated quite a bit but that she still had a lot of pain. She also stated that she had not been able to follow the detoxification program outlined by her dentist to reduce her total mercury body burden. She said her stomach was so sensitive from having taken aspirin for so many years that she couldn't take any vitamin C. As a result she could not take the cysteine either. This fact has been brought to the attention of her dentist who will try to work up a protocol that she can follow.

In closing this chapter on anecdotal experiences I would like to quote two additional case histories. These will be quoted in their entirety exactly as published. Please take special note of the dates of these articles as they serve to reinforce the fact that the problem is certainly not new.

This case was published in Dental Cosmos, Vol. XIII, 1871, pages 637–638.

MISCELLANY
ABSTRACTS AND SELECTIONS
By J. W. WHITE

Dental Times

Dr. Elihum R. Pettit gives a case in practice, showing the "Injurious Effects of Amalgam."

"On October 1st, 1868, I inserted a large amalgam filling in the second inferior left molar, mesial and grinding surfaces. On the 8th of the same month the patient, Mrs. P. ate two or three fried oysters and almost immediately afterward became very sick at the stomach—without vomiting, however, but with a rash breaking out upon her face and neck, with itching, and oedema of the face and eyelids. But the next day she was quite well, except that the rash had not entirely disappeared. About a month afterward, again partaking of oysters, the same symptoms returned, with coldness of the extremities, to such a degree as to become alarming. Attributing these symptoms to the oysters, she abstained from them entirely.

"On the 17th of May, 1870, I applied the arsenical paste to the pulp of the right inferior second molar tooth of the same patient, in the usual manner. About an hour later, after the lady had returned to her home, the symptoms above mentioned reappeared. She returned the next day, when I cleaned out the cavity and removed the pulp. The rash had then partially disappeared. On the succeeding day, the 19th, when she returned to have the tooth filled she complained of all her teeth being sore, and some of them slightly loose, but especially those on the right side of the mouth and in the immediate neighborhood of the tooth to the pulp of which the paste had been applied. The rash had also returned in a greater degree than before. I am quite confident that the patient could not have swallowed any of the paste, although the cavity was on the proximal surface and the tooth was properly protected by napkins, so that these effects must have been produced entirely by the absorption of the arsenious acid through the pulp. The patient left the city the same day, the 19th, and while absent the same symptoms were produced by fish and radishes.

"The similarity of these symptoms with those produced

long before by the oyster point to the same cause for both, as there had previously been no idiosyncrasy in regard to any article of food. Upon careful examination no cause could be discovered why such effects should be produced, when, to test the matter, I removed the amalgam filling, supposing that the mercury might have produced and kept up such a state of irritability in the system that articles of food, which might have even a slight tendency to disagree with her, even if not sufficient to be noticed, might produce such alarming results. Since that time (May, 1870), there has been no return of the symptoms, although she has partaken freely of oysters and such other food as before disagreed with her, thus proving these effects to have been caused by the mercury.

"Although such cases are rare, they are sufficiently frequent to cause us to be on our guard against them, while they should lead us to discard from our practice, wherever it is possible to do so, a substance so insidiously deleterious in its effects. They should lead us also to remove all amalgam from the teeth of any of our patients, who may have been suffering from ill health from any obscure or uncertain cause, which will not yield to the ordinary remedies; while those who are in the habit of inserting such fillings generally, making gold the exception, incur a responsibility which few, who are aware of such cases, would care to assume."

The second article appeared in the Periscope section of The Dental Cosmos, Vol. XVI, 1874, pages 213–214.

"POISONING FROM CORROSIVE SUBLIMATE GENERATED IN THE MOUTH FROM AMALGAM PLUGS IN THE TEETH—Having been invited by an eminent gentleman of the medical profession to attend a convention of the State Medical Society to submit to its consideration a matter of vital importance to the human family, and being unable to comply with the invitation, I have written this article to lay the matter before the medical profession and ask its cooperation.

The matter which I wished to bring to the notice of the profession is the poisoning of thousands of people all over the world from corrosive sublimate generated in the mouth from amalgam plugs in the teeth. Neither Asiatic cholera, nor smallpox, nor any malarious disease is doing half the mischief in the world that is being done by this poisoning. Every medical man of any considerable practice has undoubtedly had numerous cases of it, but never knew what it was. The symptoms are so numerous and varied in different cases that it would be impossible to give them all in this short article, but I will say that a person is liable to be treated for dyspepsia, neuralgia, paralysis, consumption, and numerous throat-diseases. The patient gradually wastes away as if going into a decline, and no medicine will afford any relief. In many cases the difficulty steals on so gently as not to excite the least alarm, and continues very gradually for a number of years till the patient becomes a total wreck; while in others the attack comes on violently, and the friends and attending physician think the patient is dying; but he will again rally, and again be prostrated.

There is such a resemblance in the symptoms to nearly all the diseases to which human flesh is heir that the physician is led to treat the patient for some disease which seems to be a very clear case, but his patient gets worse. In more than twenty cases that I have had, nearly all had been pronounced by some physician as having consumption. In nearly all the cases there are at times a very bad cough, eyes sunken, and haggard expression and deep blue or dark color under the eyes, invariably a metallic taste in the mouth, water flowing from the mouth in the night while asleep so as to wet the pillow, and in most cases extreme prostration.

I have not time now to detail the manner in which the corrosive sublimate is formed in the mouth, further than to say that the quicksilver in the plugs is driven off by the heat of the mouth in very minute particles, and, combining with the chlorine in the fluids of the mouth, or any saline substance, such as our food, passes into the stomach, and produces slow poisoning. If the State Medical Society will appoint a committee to visit this place, I will show them several cases that will place the matter beyond controversy.

There are some twelve thousand dentists in the United States doing a wholesale business at this poisoning, and I ask the cooperation of the State Medical Society, as guardians of the public health, to assist in getting an act of Congress passed making it a penitentiary offense to place any poisonous substance in teeth that will injure the people.—J. Payne, D.D.S., in Chicago Medical Journal.''

Sound familiar? Science has progressed light years since that article appeared in 1874 but has anything changed? The recommendations made by Dr. Payne in 1874 are just as valid today as they were then. Professionals talking to professionals will not change the situation. The only way the problem will ever be solved is for the general public, the recipients of mercury amalgam fillings, to raise their voices to a level that Congress and the Establishment can recognize. Which, unfortunately in this day and age of vested interests, has to be pretty loud.

Chapter 10 provides a list of actions you can take to help bring an end to this 150 year old war.

WHAT HAS CHANGED SINCE ORIGINAL PUBLICATION OF THIS BOOK?

Chapter 10 through 14 that follow contain new or revised data since first publication. The decision was made to utilize this format rather than updating individual chapters so that readers would be able to readily see the magnitude of additional scientific data being presented.

Although some of the subjects contained in these new chapters have been previously covered to some extent in the 1st edition of the book, the information now being presented either augments and expands on the original material or reflects entirely new or different data, research or events.

Further, there is one other aspect of this revision of which I would like to inform you. In the original manuscript I attempted to be objective and impartial, presenting both sides of the story so that the reader could make up his own mind about the issue. The events that have transpired since that time make it extremely difficult for me to remain impartial. I am referring primarily to the complete inability of the Amalgamites (those claiming amalgam is safe and advocating its continued use as the dental material of choice) to present one shred of acceptable scientific data supporting their position. More importantly, their descent into the realm of dirty tricks, character assassination, restraint of trade, suppression of individual civil rights, and the publication in certain magazines or other media of undocumented, referenced articles containing unsupportable statements, as a means of attempting to sway public opinion and defend their pro-amalgam position is inexcusable.

The above considerations not withstanding, I will not lower my standards or deviate from the original intent of this book. By presenting only scientific data, you the reader, can be the final judge and jury.

Sam Ziff
September 1986

CHAPTER 10

THE UNSAFETY OF AMALGAM

An international "Workshop on the Biocompatibility of Metals in Dentistry", sponsored by the National Institute of Dental Research (NIDR) and hosted by the ADA was held at ADA Headquarters in Chicago, Illinois July 11-13, 1984. A transcript of the Workshop was prepared and published by the ADA later that year.

The Workshop resulted in some modification of the standard ADA policy statements regarding amalgam: 1) For the first time, the ADA publicly admitted that mercury vapor is released from amalgam fillings during function (chewing) and 2) That blood and urine analysis for mercury content or levels in these biological fluids does not correspond to toxicity. However, although admitting to the release of mercury vapor, the ADA qualified their position by also saying that the amount of mercury vapor released is so small that it could not be considered a health hazard except in those few individuals who may have developed mercury hypersensitivity. Moreover, the incidence of such mercury hypersensitivity is estimated to be less than 1% of the population.

There are two aspects of the ADA position statement that are very disturbing: 1) There is no scientific data to support their statements that the amount of mercury vapor released could not constitute a health hazard. In fact, quite the contrary happens to be the accepted scientific position, i.e. the minimum toxic dose of mercury for humans is not known. 2) Their use of an estimate that less than 1% of the population is hypersensitive to mercury is totally without scientific foundation. If the "less than 1%" figure is not based on scientific fact, then on what is it based? Nobody seems to know exactly where the 1% figure came from but an ADA spokesman stated in a recent public forum that he thought it originated during a question and answer session at the July 1984 Workshop and was the opinion of one of the presenters based on his own personal experiences.

Through its testing, certification and advertising programs the ADA spends a great deal of money, time and effort on creating and projecting an image of credibility, authority and "protector of the people". So when someone sees the ADA seal of approval on a product they almost automatically accept that as primary proof that it is safe. The same can be said for public policy announcements made by the ADA.

Consequently, when the ADA makes public pronouncements that amalgam is safe, that the amount of mercury vapor being released cannot harm you, and that less than 1% of the population are hypersensitive to mercury, a great majority of the public exposed to such statements is going to believe them without questioning whether or not they are true. Unfortunately, because so many of our dentists and physicians are never exposed to any scientific literature to the contrary, they also tend to go along with the ADA statements without ever questioning them.

Is there scientific research that presents data that can be considered contrary to the position taken by the ADA and the NIDR? Lets look at the facts presently available:

In 1967 L. Magos, in a set of experiments with mice, demonstrated that mercury vapor in its elemental form can reach the brain. Mercury vapor inhaled into the lungs has an absorption rate of 70% to 100%. Further, the total time for blood to make one complete circulation in the body is 15–18 seconds. Therefore, it is a question of seconds and not hours in evaluating whether mercury in the highly diffusible elemental form can reach the brain and other organs. In its elemental form, mercury vapor readily penetrates the blood brain barrier and placental membrane.

Once inside the brain, the elemental mercury vapor is oxidized into its mercuric form. The same blood brain barrier that we assume functions to limit or restrict the brain uptake of mercury that has already been oxidized, now functions to restrict the escape of oxidized mercury from the brain. This results in a much smaller proportion of mercury being released from the brain in comparison to other organs. Thus in his experiments, Magos found that 8 days after exposure, about 8% of the body burden of mercury was in the brain.

Two other major factors that must be considered in addressing the question of whether chronic exposure to micro doses of mercury vapor being released from dental amalgam fillings have the potential to harm you are:

1) The manner in which each dose of mercury is handled by the body bears significantly on its potential to cause harm. Rothstein et al. (1964) demonstrated that each dose of mercury that is inhaled disappears with the same kinetics (movement) as in single-exposure experiments. Distribution of repeated doses is determined by the time elapsing between the individual exposures. In other words, each individual dose of mercury behaves independently in the body with regard to absorption, turnover, deposition in tissue, and excretion. These kinetics of mercury were also confirmed by Magos in his 1967 experiment related above.

2) The other factor that is so important, in evaluating the potential of mercury to harm, relates to how the body gets rid of mercury. Rothstein and Hayes (1960) in experiments utilizing rats, demonstrated that there were three phases in the clearance of mercury. There was a rapid phase, a slower phase and the important discovery of a third and much slower phase. This slowest phase represented about 15% of the original dose and was characterized by a half-time of 100 days. Scientists have since postulated that the presence of the slowest component would cause accumulation over the life of the animal in cases of chronic exposure.

M. Sugita (1978) looked at the biological half-times of heavy metals, not by experimentally injecting doses of heavy metals, but by autopsy studies of inhabitants of the Tokyo area of Japan who had experienced no known exposure to an abnormally high level of heavy metals and who had died sudden deaths by accident. The biological half-times were obtained by observation of the amounts accumulated naturally in human organs and tissues according to age.

Sugita concluded that the biological half-time of the slowest component in humans would be 18 to 20 years in the cerebrum (forebrain and midbrain–the largest part of the brain). Citing other researchers, Sugita brings up evidence supporting the existence of the third and slowest component indicating that when the dose is large the biological half-time is short, but when the dose is small, the biological half-time is long.

In a 1984 paper, Bernard and Purdue developed metabolic compartmental models for methyl and inorganic mercury and state that for both methylmercury and inorganic mercury a half-life of 10,000 days would be appropriate for the slowest component. (10,000 days equates to over 27 years) In discussing inorganic mercury the authors state that the major route of human exposure to metallic mercury is by inhalation of mercury vapor.

What is the significance of these extremely long half-times for mercury in the brain in relation to the release of mercury vapor from amalgam dental fillings? Two recently published autopsy studies show positive correlations between the numbers and surfaces of amalgam dental fillings and mercury content of the brain.

The first was a study by Schiele et al. that was presented at a Symposium titled "Amalgam–Viewpoint from medicine and dental medicine", held in Cologne, West Germany, March 12, 1984. Dr. Schiele and his colleagues did autopsy studies on 44 persons who had died suddenly. The studies were carried out in the forensic department of the University of Erlangen-Nurnberg. There were 25 males and 19 females in the study ranging in age between 16 and 57 years of age. The brains and kidneys of these accident victims were evaluated for mercury content. The researchers found a clear correlation between the number and surfaces of silver amalgam fillings and the mercury content of the brain and kidneys. The researchers were also able to determine that there was a correlation between age and mercury content in the brain. However, they could find no correlation between sex, place of residence, occupation, smoking, condition of fillings and the number of gold restorations.

The second study was done at the Karolinski Institute, National Institute of Environmental Medicine, Stockholm, Sweden. The study was done in the Department of Hygiene which is headed by Professor Lars Friberg (one of the world's foremost research authorities on mercury) and was published in the Swedish Medicine Journal LAKARTIDNINGEN (1986).

Studies on autopsy material from 17 individuals (dead by accident) have shown that mercury in the central nervous system can be related to the number of amalgam fillings in the mouth. Results from analysis of occipital lobe cortex, cerebellar cortex and ganglion semilunare for total mercury, shows on average a higher concentration in the cortex when the number of amalgam fillings is large compared to when the number is lower. The research team also developed a method of differentiating between different types of mercury. This was done to see if the mercury they found was coming from the food chain or from the amalgam fillings. The two types of mercury have different half-times in the brain. Methylmercury usually the type present in our food chain, is reduced to half in70 days whereas inorganic mercury (elemental mercury vapor) coming from amalgam has a half-time of more than 20 years in some parts of the brain. People with amalgam fillings have the same amount of methylmercury but about three (3) times more inorganic mercury compared to those without amalgam fillings.

When a Swedish newspaper interviewed Dr. Magnus Nylander, a member of the research team on the above autopsy study, he was quoted as saying: "There is still much research to be done. We do not know if the levels we have found are dangerous. There are no permissible limits on this. But it is known that mercury is one of the most poisonous substances known."

The above statement by Dr. Nylander gets right to the heart of the mercury/amalgam filling issue and differs from the irresponsible statement issued by the ADA advising the American public that there is no reason to be concerned about the small amount of mercury vapor being released from dental amalgam fillings. Stated another way, THERE IS NO SCIENTIFIC RESEARCH INDICATING OR PROVING THAT THE LEVELS OF MERCURY BEING FOUND IN THE BRAINS OF HUMANS CAN BE CONSIDERED SAFE. NOR IS THERE RESEARCH SHOWING THAT THERE HAS BEEN NO BRAIN DAMAGE ASSOCIATED WITH ITS PRESENCE.

It is obvious from the above, regardless of the thousands of scientific studies already published on the harmful effects of mercury, that our present knowledge of the relationship of these effects to acknowledged disease conditions is very limited. For example, I would like to quote from an 1983 Medical Text Book "Environmental and Occupational Medicine": "The spinal fluid in humans exposed occupationally to inorganic mercury contains measurable concentrations of mercury. In 20 exposed subjects, 3 with overt clinical evidence of mercurialism, detectable amounts of mercury were found in the spinal fluid of 65 percent, ranging from a trace up to 8.5 ug/L." (micrograms per liter)

How many debilitating health conditions or diseases can be related to, or may be associated with, impairment of normal neurologic or bio-chemical functions of the Central Nervous System (CNS)? What part, if any, do mercury or other heavy metals play in such disease processes? Are one or more of these heavy metals involved in such diseases as Alzheimer's, Amyotrophic Lateral Sclerosis, Systemic Lupus Erythematosis and multi-factoral syndromes such as Multiple Sclerosis, etc.?

Although some research, such as that related above, has demonstrated the presence of mercury in the brain, nerves, and spinal fluid; and other studies have identified the capability of mercury to inhibit various enzyme systems involved in the normal function of these tissues and fluids, there is almost a total lack of scientific data or studies investigating if mercury is a possible causative factor. However, you must admit that the possibility that heavy metals may be involved in the initiation of these conditions, which are afflicting humans at an ever increasing rate, is indeed an exciting prospect and challenge for medicine and science to address.

When we talk about elemental mercury vapor you should also be aware of what some of the world's foremost experts on mercury think. The following statement is quoted from a 1980 World Health Organization (WHO) publication titled "Recommended Health-Based Limits in Occupational Exposure to Heavy Metals: "The most hazardous forms of mercury to human health are elemental mercury vapor and the short-chain alkylmercurials". The authors of the 1980 report also refer to a 1976 WHO report titled "Mercury: Environmental Health Criteria 1" which states: "The primary biochemical lesions associated with mercury poisoning have not been established. Virtually nothing is known of the biochemical disturbances associated with exposure to metallic mer-

cury vapor". THESE STATEMENTS BY RESPONSIBLE SCI-
ENTISTS TREAT THIS INSIDIOUS POISON WITH DUE
RESPECT.

In this same context, I think the public would have been
better served if the author of the article titled "The Mercury Scare"
which appeared in the March 1986 issue of *Consumer Reports*,
had taken a more responsible position and investigated the scientific data involved in the mercury/amalgam issue rather than publish a totally biased and one sided article that resorted to smear
tactics and character assassination rather than scientific data to
support the pro-amalgam views of the author.

The author of this report was Assistant Editor Larry Katzenstein. Mr. Katzenstein called and talked to me in January 1986
prior to publication of the article. It was apparent during the short
conversation I had with Mr. Katzenstein that he wasn't interested
in any of the scientific facts related to the amalgam controversy.
The only question he asked me related to whether I had obtained a
degree in nutrition from Donsbach University in California. When
I asked him if he had read my book *The Toxic Time Bomb*, he
replied that he had not. I then advised him that I had in my
possession over 1400 scientific articles dealing with the toxicology
of mercury and that I would be happy to provide him with any
scientific data he might need for his article, he replied that he had
all the information he needed to complete his article.

Why the Managing Editor of *Consumer Reports* would permit such a slanted article to be printed on such an important
public health issue presents some very interesting ethical questions.

Before I leave the *Consumer Reports* article, I have to confess
that I was somewhat amazed that Dr. Thomas W. Clarkson would
even consent to participate in the type of forum presented by
Consumer Reports. Dr. Clarkson is a world renowned researcher
on mercury who has published many important scientific papers
on the subject. Most recently, he was the principle author of the
United States Environmental Protection Agency (EPA— report
titled "Mercury Health Effects Update, Health Issue Assessment".
In paragraph 2.1.1, page 2-2 of this report Dr. Clarkson states that
the total daily intake of mercury from all sources should not
exceed 30 micrograms of mercury for a 70 kilogram body weight.

Taking into consideration estimates of average daily dietary intakes, the report states that to restrict total intake to 30 micrograms of mercury per 70 kilogram of body weight, the average mercury intake from air would have to be limited to 20 micrograms of mercury per 70 kilograms of body weight. To maintain this level, the air would have to contain an average concentration of no more than 1 microgram of mercury per cubic meter of air, assuming inhalation of 20 cubic meters a day by the 70 kilogram adult.

What Dr. Clarkson has stated here is that the average environmental level of mercury in the atmosphere should not exceed 1 microgram per cubic meter. Yet, this is the same Dr. Clarkson who is quoted in *Consumer Reports* as saying that a mercury-vapor analyzer can't answer the question of how much mercury vapor gets absorbed by the body tissues. I wonder how Dr. Clarkson intends for the EPA to monitor and determine the atmospheric mercury content?

From the statements attributed to Dr. Clarkson I would have to assume that he was not aware of, or perhaps he chose to ignore all of the research showing the routine release of elemental mercury vapor from amalgam fillings at levels that have the potential to greatly exceed the EPA standard he helped establish. It also seems apparent that not only is Dr. Clarkson not currently giving the proper respect to this vast array of research, but he did the same thing in 1984 when he wrote the EPA report. On page 3-20 of the report he states: "The atmosphere is the only source of human exposure to Hg° (elemental mercury vapor)." What makes that statement so puzzling is that I have personal knowledge that Dr. Clarkson was made aware of the research and the controversy regarding the release of mercury from amalgam dental fillings.

I have no idea of what has motivated Dr. Clarkson to take the position reflected in the Mercury Scare article. However, some of his statements in the article appear to be in conflict and even contrary to data contained in some of his previously published scientific papers. For example the following paragraphs are quoted from the Mercury Scare article: "Clarkson told CU that a person's mercury exposure can best be assessed by measuring the mercury levels in blood and urine. The urine level provides the best measure of "body burden," or long-term exposure to mercury, while the blood level reflects recent exposure." . . . "Almost every-one, Clarkson said, has detectable levels of mercury in the urine and blood. The main source of mercury in most people's bodies is the food they eat, seafood in particular. Clarkson expressed sur-prise that the CU reporter, who eats tuna at lunch most days, had such modest mercury levels in his blood and urine."

It would seem to me that the second quotation expressing surprise at the reporter's low mercury blood and urine levels in spite of ingesting so much sea food daily, brings into serious ques-tion the validity of the first quotation stating that urine levels provide the best measure of body burden. Aside from the fact that most scientists have concluded that mercury urine is a poor indica-tor of toxicity, there has been no valid threshold established for mercury. Moreover, the time of day that a urine sample is taken has a bearing on the amount of mercury that will be present in the urine. This is called the diurnal variation. In a recent report, Calder et al. (1984) demonstrated that the urine mercury concen-tration was highest in the morning and lowest in the evening. It would also appear that Dr. Clarkson is ignoring the vast amount of research data, some of which was quoted previously, establish-ing the existence of a very slow phase of mercury excretion. The principle of the slow phase is that chronic exposure to micro doses of mercury will cause the continued accumulation in various organs over the lifetime of the individual. A fact which has been confirmed by autopsy studies.

Now, I am not a scientist, but I don't think you can have it both ways. By that I mean that I don't believe you can assay urine for mercury being excreted by the body and at the same time state that low levels of mercury in the urine means that the body isn't accumulating and storing mercury when there is so much scientific data indicating that it is being retained and stored. This was most aptly expressed by Casser-Pullicino et al. (1985), who concluded their study with the following comment: "Moreover the blood and urinary mercury levels show little or no correlation with the mani-festation of mercurialism. There appears to be no level above which symptoms can be expected, or below which symptoms can-not occur."

As Dr. Clarkson also mentions the importance of blood mer-cury levels I would just like to bring to your attention the conclusion of another recent study, Snapp K. R., Svare C. W. and Peterson L. C. (1985): "This study showed there was a reduction in blood mercury levels when existing dental amalgam restorations were removed and replaced with a nonmercury containing restorative material."

Since original publications of *The Toxic Time Bomb*, there have been several scientific studies published confirming and expanding on the release of mercury vapor from mercury/amalgam dental fillings under various conditions.

In March 1985, Emler and Cardone of Oral Roberts Univeristy reported their study titled "An Assessment of Mercury in Mouth Air". What is so important about this study is that the subjects were all pediatric dental patients ages 5–12. These children had low exposure to mercury, low fish intake, and no alcohol intake (this affects how the body handles mercury). The mouth air mercury levels were compared before and after the insertion of an amalgam restoration. The report concluded with this statement: "Dental amalgam restorations and mercury vapor exposure were shown to be causally related. Chewing increased the evaporation of mercury from one week old dental amalgams."

In April 1985, Patterson et al. published a study titled "Mercury in Human Breath from Dental Amalgam". These workers confirmed Dr. Svare's findings that chewing stimulated the release of mercury vapor from amalgam fillings. They then went on to demonstrate the same or higher release of mercury vapor from amalgam fillings after tooth brushing for one minute with a soft tooth brush and a commercial tooth paste. Dr. Patterson and his colleagues make the following statement in their report: "We report here the results of our measurements of mercury vapor concentrations in the exhaled breath of 172 persons, a few of which exceed probable safe exposure limits and appear high enough to be a chronic toxicologic hazard for some people with numerous amalgam fillings."

In August 1985, Drs. Vimy and Lorscheider published a classic study which, instead of measuring exhaled air as in the other studies, measured the mercury vapor concentrations of intra-oral air (in the mouth) before and after chewing gum for 10 minutes. Their study also revealed that once you stopped chewing it took another 90 minutes before the intra-oral mercury vapor readings returned to their pre-stimulation level. This data was then extrapolated for three meals and two snacks a day and a series of formulae were developed that computed the potential accrued increase in mercury body burden that would be directly attributable to dental amalgam fillings. The authors make the following statement: "These mercury dosages from dental amalgam were as much as 18-fold the allowable daily limits established by some countries for mercury exposure from all sources in the environment. The results demonstrate that the amount of elemental mercury released from dental amalgam exceeds or comprises a major percentage of internationally accepted threshold limit values for environmental mercury exposure. It is concluded that dental amalgam mercury makes a major contribution to total daily dose."

Dr. Bengt Fredin, a researcher at Lund University in Sweden, in a recently completed study (submitted for publication) determined that the ingestion of hot liquids (soup, coffee, tea, etc.) also stimulated the release of mercury vapor from dental amalgam fillings the same as chewing or tooth brushing.

In addition to the above studies, there are several other in vitro studies that have been published that were designed to demonstrate and record the amount of mercury vapor released from different types of amalgams under various conditions of age, temperature, saliva (natural and artificial) and wear. All show the release of mercury vapor in varying amounts under different conditions.

What all of this data means, is that irrefutable scientific evidence exists demonstrating the release of mercury vapor from amalgam dental fillings under a wide range of natural conditions and functions. If there is a failing in all of this scientific effort, it is that no one has as yet put all the data together showing what the collective and cumulative total of all this mercury vapor being released would be on a daily basis. For example, what would be the daily intake for a person of average weight and height, who had approximately 12 amalgam surfaces, and brushed his teeth twice a day, ate three meals and two snacks a day, drank three cups of hot liquids during the day, chewed gum an average of one hour a day and who also routinely drank one or two soft drinks a day?

Taking into consideration the amount released during direct stimulation as well as the 60–90 minute period of continued release of mercury vapor after stimulation, and the fact that most researchers have indicated in their articles that the release from the individual activity on which they were reporting could, in some instances, exceed present threshold values. It does not seem unreasonable to conclude that some individuals are going to be chronically inhaling mercury vapor at levels that will routinely be in the toxic range for that individual.

This also means that, for some people, the contribution of mercury vapor from amalgam dental fillings alone could equal or exceed the maximum allowable daily intake from all sources (dietary, water, atmosphere) of 30 micrograms of mercury for a 70 kilogram body weight established by the E.P.A. (70 kilograms equate to about 154 pounds). An interesting question would be: What happens to the 110 pound woman, with a mouth full of amalgam fillings that produce 30 micrograms of mercury vapor per day? Will she be at greater risk? What is she is pregnant, what is happening biochemically to the fetus? Or, what about children who at very early ages/weights can have the same level of exposure as adults?

In the face of such overwhelming scientific evidence demonstrating the release of mercury vapor, what are the ADA, NIDR and the rest of the pro-amalgam advocates doing to counter it?

Believe it or not, they are using the *Consumer Reports* "Mercury Scare" article and an article authored by Dr. Robert S. Baratz that appeared in The Harvard Medical School Health Letter, Vol XI, No. 1, November 1985 to satisfy requests for information. More tragically, many ADA pro-amalgam dentists have had these articles reproduced and have them in their reception rooms.

The Harvard Medical Letter article, as the one in *Consumer Reports*, does not cite any scientific reference to support any of the allegations made by the author. The article is titled "Mercury in Dental Fillings: Is There a Problem?" Dr. Baratz in 2 1/2 pages attempts to impugn all of the scientific articles published in refereed dental and medical journals dealing with the release of mercury from dental amalgam fillings.

His approach is certainly novel and original because he claims that the instrument used to measure the mercury vapor in these studies was an industrial machine not designed to measure mercury vapor accurately under the conditions present in the oral cavity. To give you some idea of the magnitude of his position I would like to quote one paragraph: "Very small amounts of mercury do escape from our fillings, but only under forced conditions with high and continuous friction. The rate of release is at least one thousand times, and probably a million times, slower that the estimates obtained from industrial air-sampling machines, and these rates are only sustained for a few minutes."

So there you have it, in one paragraph Dr. Baratz in effect is saying that scientific findings derived from valid scientific experiments and studies performed at the University of Calgary Medical School, Oral Roberts University Dental School, Lund University in Sweden, University of Iowa Dental School, and two facilities in New Zealand in addition to scientific articles dealing with the engineering validity of gold foil mercury vapor analyzers are all flawed and invalid. It would be extremely interesting to see if Dr. Baratz, who evidently considers himself an expert on this subject, could get the same article published in a refereed scientific journal.

The Editor of The Harvard Medical School Health Letter is William I. Bennett, M.D. I have in my possession a letter written by Dr. Bennett, in response to an irate reader's letter, in which he makes the following statement: "We do not accept your charge of bias. The Health Letter does not feel an obligation to present all sides of an issue equally. We take responsibility for weighing the credibility of various sides and choosing among them. In the case of the article on dental amalgam, the editors and advisory board of the Health Letter accepted Dr. Baratz's account of the situation."

In two biased and undocumented articles replete with sarcasm and innuendo, the pro-amalgam advocates have reached hundreds of thousands of innocent readers, unfamiliar with the subject or aware that there is another side to be heard. As a direct result these reader's will not question the continued implantation of a poison in their mouths or request medical consideration of mercury toxicity as a possible cause of their existing health problems.

These two articles embody the following basic arguments used by the Amalgamites to counter the overwhelming array of scientific evidence indicating that a serious and potentially dangerous condition exists related to dental amalgam fillings: Most of the research is flawed because:

1) Most people breathe through their nose when chewing thereby bypassing any mercury vapor that may be in their mouths. These critics also seem to totally overlook the fact that the Vimy and Lorscheider research reflects due consideration of the oral/ nasal breathing ratios as reflected in existing scientific literature. They also totally ignore the work of Patrick Stortebecker, M.D., Ph.D. a world renowned Neurologist who has scientifically demonstrated the direct passage of mercury from the mouth to the brain via either, an open venous (valve-less) communication between the tooth-pulp, the bone-marrow of the jaws and the intra-cranial cavity with the brain, or direct oro-nasal cranial venous pathways or by the olfactory nerves or the trigeminal nerves.

2) The instrument used to measure the intra-oral mercury vapor levels is not designed to be used for that purpose. It is designed to measure mercury vapor in the atmosphere and in industrial work environments and can be off as much as 1000% if used in the mouth. The instrument in question is the Jerome Mercury Vapor Analyzer and these amalgam champions and ADA spokesmen don't offer any scientific documentation to support their indictment of this state-of-the-art instrument accepted by governments and scientists all over the world as the standard for measuring mercury vapor.

When viewing the tremendous amount of scientific research casting serious doubts on the safety of dental amalgam a basic question concerning the pro-amalgam organizations and individuals involved demands consideration. Why are they fighting so hard to defend their right to implant a poison in your body in the fact of overwhelming scientific evidence contraindicating such action?

This also leads us to question the true intent and motives of the NIDR and ADA when large amounts of taxpayers dollars are expended to host international workshops and symposia to develop recommendations concerning future research that will help insure the biocompatibility of materials used in dentistry which, for all intents and purposes, are then ignored in the awarding of research grants. For example, the following future research recommendations were the product of the NIDR/ADA Workshop on Biocompatibility of Metals in Dentistry (July 1984):

1. Diagnostic and analytical procedures should be investigated for documenting exposure to metals in alloys.

2. An evaluation should be made of nickel salts or other nickel compounds which may be formed during the fabrication and use of base-metal alloys.

3. Investigate the role of nickel, beryllium and chromium as potential carcinogens in dental laboratory technicians.

4. An assessment should be made of mercury loss from chewing on dental amalgams of different alloy compositions.

5. Studies should be initiated to determine whether methyl mercury can be formed in vivo.

6. Epidemiologic studies should be initiated to assess the prevalence of mercury allergy in the United States population.

7. Biological sampling procedures should be investigated to determine a reliable means of estimating body burden of mercury.

8. Studies should be initiated to accurately assess blood levels of mercury which may result from dental amalgam.

9. Research should be initiated to determine whether the effects of mercury on T-lymphocytes may be a means of early detection of subclinical manifestations of mercury toxicity.

10. Studies should be initiated to develop more definitive tests for determining the hypersensitivity to metals used in dentistry.

11. Studies should examine the potential that thyroid gland enlargement may be an early predictor of mercury intoxication.

12. Studies are encouraged to determine whether a relationship exists between maternal exposure to mercury and teratogenesis.

13. The effects of conditions which accelerate corrosion of dental materials on the release of metal ions should be studied in more detail.

14. The composition of corrosion products should be identified as well as the effect they may have on oral tissues.

15. Continued research is recommended on the development of alternative restorative materials.

With the exception of recommendation #13 on which millions of dollars have already been expended, I consider the recommended areas of research to be excellent. The proper design, funding, and execution or completion of research projects in support of the above recommendations could resolve the entire mercury/amalgam controversy. This aspect alone should have warranted priority and special consideration to insure appropriate projects were submitted for funding. Unfortunately, the realities of the situation are that, although two years have elapsed since the Workshop, almost nothing has been done to fund recommended areas of research critical to resolving the controversy.

On May 12, 1986 I wrote a letter to Dr. Harold Loe, Director of the Institute of Dental Research requesting the status of the Workshop future research recommendations. On May 23, 1986 I received a reply complete with two computer listings of grants awarded during FY 1985 and FY 1986 totalling $18,159,017.00 and $20,190,619.00 respectively. Of this total of more than 38 million dollars I could only identify three projects in FY 1985 ($112,639) and two projects in FY 1986 ($162,865) that addressed the Workshop recommendations dealing with the release of mercury from amalgam fillings or it's biocompatibility.

Are you fascinated by the mind boggling figure of $38,000,000.00? Then how about $88,380,000.00? Yes, that is correct 88 million three hundred and eighty thousand dollars. That is the total amount of funds expended on dental research by the NIDR during FY 1984. I have no problem with the allocation of funds for dental research. What I have a problem with is the fact that of that total amount of research dollars, only $48,958 was expended on research investigating the biocompatibility of dental silver amalgam fillings. This information is contained in a letter signed by James O. Mason, M.D., Dr. P.H., Acting Assistant Secretary for Health and dated May 28, 1985. The letter goes on to say that "So far in FY 1985, the Institute has expended $83,494 in this area. It is expected that this amount will increase significantly during FY 1986."

Based on the project data that was provided, it is apparent that no forceful action is being taken by responsible government agencies to fund the research and seriously investigate the biocompatibility of mercury amalgam dental fillings.

REFERENCES

1. NIDR/ADA Workshop on Biocompatibility of Metals in Dentistry, July 11-13, 1984, Chicago, IL. Transcript available from ADA.

2. NIDR/Workshop: Biocompatibility of Metals in Dentistry. Journal of the American Dental Association, Vol. 109, issue 3:469-471, Nov. 1984.

3. Magos L. Mercury-blood interaction and mercury uptake by the brain after exposure. Environmental Research Vol. 1:323-337, 1967.

4. Rothstein A. and Hayes A.D. The turnover of mercury in rats exposed repeatedly to inhalation of vapor. Health Physics Vol. 10:1099-1113, 1964.

5. Rothstein A. and Hayes A.D. The metabolism of mercury in the rat studied by isotope techniques. Journal of Pharmacology and Experimental Therapeutics Vol. 130:166-176, 1960.

6. Sugita M. The biological half-time of heavy metals. International Archives of Occupational and Environmental Health, Vol. 41:25-40, 1978.

7. Schiele R. et al. Studies on the mercury content in brain and kidney related to number and condition of amalgam fillings. Institute of Occupational and Social Medicine. Univeristy of Erlangen-Nurnberg. Symposium March 12, 1984, Cologne, Germany. Amalgam — Viewpoints From Medicine and Dental Medicine.

8. Friberg L., Kullman L., Birger L. and Nylander M. Mercury in the central nervous system in relation to amalgam fillings. LAKARTIDNINGEN Vol. 83, Issue 7:519-521, 1986.

9. Mercury from dental fillings is spread to the brain and accumulates Svenska Dagbladet Feb 4, 1985. (Interview with Dr. Nylander translated by Dr. Mats Hanson)

10. Bernard S.R. and Purdue P. Metabolic models for methyl and inorganic mercury. Health Physics, Vol. 46, Issue 3:695-699, 1984.

11. Recommended Health-Based Limits in Occupational Exposure to Heavy Metals. Page 102, Technical Report Series 647, WHO, Geneva, 1980.

12. Battigelli M.C. Mercury, In: Environmental and Occupational Medicine, Little, Brown and Co., Boston, 1983. Chapter 39, page 454.

13. The mercury scare. Consumer Reports, Vol. 51, No. 3:151-153, March, 1986.

14. Clarkson T.W. Mercury Health Effects Update. Health Issue Assessment, EPA-600/8-84-019F, August 1984, Final Report.

15. Clarkson T.W. The pharmacology of mercury compounds. Annual Reviews of Pharmacology, Vol. 12:375-406, 1972.

16. Calder I.M. et al. Diurnal variations in urinary mercury excretion. Human Toxicology, Vol. 3:463-467, 1984.

17. Cassar-Pullicino V.N. et al. Multiple metallic mercury emboli. The British Journal of Radiology, Vol. 58:470-474, 1985.

18. Snapp K.R. et al. Contribution of dental amalgam to blood mercury levels. Journal of Dental Research, Vol. 65 Special Issue, page 311, Abstract #1276, March 1985.

19. Emler B.F. and Cardone M. Sr. An assessment of mercury in mouth air. Journal of Dental Research, Vol. 64:247, Abstract 652, 1985.

20. Patterson J.E., Weissberg B.G. and Dennison P.J. Mercury in human breath from dental amalgams. Bull. Environ. Contam. Toxicol. Vol. 34:549-468, 1985.

21. Vimy M.J. and Lorscheider F.L. Intra-oral air mercury released from dental amalgam. Journal of Dental Research, Vol. 64:1069-1071, 1985a.

22. Vimy M.J. and Lorscheider F.L. Serial measurements of intra-oral air mercury: Estimation of daily dose from dental amalgam. Journal of Dental Research, Vol. 64:1072-1075, 1985b.

23. Baratz R.S. Mercury in dental fillings: Is there a problem? The Harvard Medical School Health Letter, Vol. XI, No. 1:5-7, Nov. 1985.

24. Stortebecker P. Mercury Poisoning from Dental Amalgam—A Hazard to Human Brain, Stortebecker Foundation for Research, Stockholm, Sweden.

CHAPTER 11

INTERNATIONAL ACADEMY OF ORAL
MEDICINE AND TOXICOLOGY (IAOMT)

In October of 1984 a group of dentists, physicians and scientists formed the International Academy of Oral Medicine and Toxicology. The statement of principle of this new organization is: "Out of concern for the health of the public at large, the Academy shall investigate the biocompatibility of oral materials and promote the informed use of those materials that are biologically acceptable."

One of the first actions taken by the Academy was to send a formal request to the ADA (Nov 30, 1984) soliciting the primary scientific documentation serving as the basis for their position that amalgam was and is a safe dental material.

In a letter dated February 19, 1985, the ADA responded to the Academy request by stating that the basis of their position was the July 11-13, 1984 NIDR/ADA "Workshop on Biocompatibility of Metals in Dentistry" which had reaffirmed the safety of dental amalgam.

As a result of the above exchange of correspondence, the IAOMT Board of Directors, at their March 1985 meeting appointed a committee to critique the transcript of the July 1984 Workshop and determine the validity of the ADA response.

The critique was completed on March 30, 1985. In April 1985

copies of the critique titled "A Critical Evaluation of the NIDR/
ADA Workshop on the Biocompatibility of Metals in Dentistry"
were mailed to the Director NIDR, President and key staff of the
ADA and the Presidents and Deans of all Colleges and Universi-
ties in the United States and Canada having Dental Schools. Permission was also granted to me to utilize portions of the document
in this Update.

As the document is 35 pages in length I have only excerpted
the Conclusions and Recommendations:

CONCLUSIONS

"The transcript of the July, 1984 NIDR/ADA Workshop presented scientific documentation establishing the following facts:

    1.   Dental amalgam is an unstable alloy that releases its com-
ponents in the form of mercury vapor, metallic ions, and abraded
particles into the oral environment.

    2.   Analytical measurements of mercury in the urine, blood,
and hair of subjects do not correlate to the body burden of toxic
effects of mercury.

    3.   The element mercury as well as a number of its com-
pounds are highly toxic to humans. In addition, it was pointed out
that other components of dental amalgam (eg. copper) are also
toxic to humans.

    4.   Mercury, as well as other metallic materials used in den-
tistry can elicit a hypersensitive (allergic) response."

**"THE WORKSHOP TRANSCRIPTS FAILED TO PRESENT
SCIENTIFIC DOCUMENTATION TO ESTABLISH THE FOL-
LOWING:**

    1.   The contribution of mercury released from dental amal-
gam to the body burden.

    2.   Minimum exposure limits resulting in pathological dam-
age to the following organs and systems in humans: brain, heart,
immune system, endocrine glands, kidney, liver, lungs, enzymes,
as well as the developing fetus.

    3.   The prevalence of mercury hypersensitivity (allergy).

    4.   Primary pathological scientific research studies verifying
the safety of the use of dental amalgam fillings in patients."

"The primary conclusion of the Workshop concerning dental

amalgam was: "On the basis of the information presented in this Workshop, there is no documented evidence for recommending the discontinuation of the use of dental amalgams as a restorative material in dentistry. Additionally, the removal of dental amalgam can only be recommended in those patients who have a true hypersensitivity to mercury or other constituents."

"The writers of this critique document have collectively reviewed over 1000 scientific articles, both primary and secondary, concerning or related to mercury, mercury toxicity, mercury hypersensitivity and amalgam. Moreover, only four primary pathological studies exist to suggest it's bioincompatibility. The frightening conclusion must be drawn that the dental profession has not encouraged the funding of primary research regarding amalgam compatibility"

"Indeed, we have been complacent enough to accept a highly methodologically flawed, statistically insignificant, and scientifically unduplicated study (Frykholm 1957) as our landmark since the late 1950's."

"The first premise of the NIDR/ADA Workshop's primary conclusion is true; –"There is no documented evidence"–. No undeniable evidence exists either for or against amalgam biocompatibility since research has not been funded. However, preliminary studies do suggest a potential health risk to patients with dental amalgams."

"Considering the toxicity of a major component of dental amalgam, (i.e., mercury) the burden of proof rests upon the scientific community, the regulatory bodies, and the dental associations which are recommending and supporting its use."

RECOMMENDATION

"Since dental amalgam contains approximately 50% by weight of mercury (a substance that is highly toxic to humans) and since the workshop failed to provide scientific evidence to substantiate the safety of dental amalgam, the International Academy of Oral Medicine and Toxicology recommends the following:

THAT THE GOVERNMENTS OF THE UNITED STATES AND CANADA DECLARE AN IMMEDIATE

PROHIBITION ON THE FURTHER USE OF DENTAL SILVER-MERCURY FILLINGS UNTIL PRIMARY SCIENTIFIC DOCUMENTATION CAN BE PROVIDED PROVING THAT THE MERCURY RELEASED FROM DENTAL FILLINGS IS NOT HARMFUL TO THE PUBLIC."

If your dentist or physician would be interested in finding out more about the International Academy of Oral Medicine and Toxicology they can write to Dr. Murray J. Vimy, #615-401 9th Ave. S.W., Calgary, Alberta, Canada T2P 3C5 or Dr. Michael Ziff, 5400 Hernandes Drive, Orlando, FL 32808.

REFERENCES

1. Vimy M.J., Ziff M. and Ziff S. A Critical Evaluation of the NIDR/ADA Workshop on Biocompatibility of Metals in Dentistry. International Academy of Oral Medicine and Toxicology, Calgary, Alberta, Canada.

CHAPTER 12

MERCURY/AMALGAM
HYPERSENSITIVITY

As indicated in Chapter 11, the official position of the ADA on this subject is that except in rare cases, individuals may develop mercury hypersensitivity or an allergic reaction from contact with mercury and it is estimated that the prevalence of mercury allergy was less than 1% of the total population.

Aside from the fact that the ADA cannot produce any scientific studies to support their position, or the fact that 1% could represent upwards of two million people, or that three of the 15 Workshop recommendations related to investigating what the incidence of hypersensitivity to mercury/amalgam actually is, let's look at what has been published in the scientific literature dealing with the subject of hypersensitivity to mercury:

1. In 1969 Djerassi and Berova found that 16.1% of their test subjects exhibited a positive reaction to amalgam and its components. What is unique about the Djerassi and Berova study, which to my knowledge has never been duplicated in any other allergy study, is that they used 60 controls who did not have any amalgam fillings in their mouths. The controls were subjected to the same series of path tests that the 180 other test subjects were given. None of the control group (without amalgam fillings) had any positive reaction to the patch tests. Conversely, 16.1% of all

the other patients in the test had a positive reaction. 22.52% of the patients whose amalgam fillings were more than five years old had a positive reaction. The greater number of patients with older amalgam fillings that reacted would appear to be further proof that mercury is escaping from these fillings and that in a great many people their body is unable to accommodate to the added burden of poison.

2.   A 1973 study by the North American Contact Dermatitis Group involving 1200 subjects demonstrated that 8% had a positive reaction to Thimerosal (Merthiolate which contains mercury) and 5% had a positive reaction to a 1% solution of Ammoniated mercury.

NOTE: Dr. A.A. Fisher, a member of the original group that conducted the above study, has recently (1985) published an article dealing with patch testing for hypersensitivity to mercury amalgam dental fillings. What I found so interesting about the article is that Dr. Fisher states: "The North American Contact Dermatitis Research Group has determined that the proper test for allergic mercury hypersensitivity is 5 percent ammoniated mercury."

The use of a 5 percent solution of ammoniated mercury is somewhat startling when compared to the 1973 study cited above which used a very dilute solution of only 1 percent ammoniated mercury. The 1973 study produced positive reactions in 65 patients or 5 percent of those tested. The immediate question that comes to mind is: If 5% of 1200 patients had a positive reaction to a mercury patch test using only a 1% solution, how many more of the 1200 participants would have reacted to a 5% solution of ammoniated mercury?

Two other aspects of this article that seem highly questionable are: 1) Dr. Fisher included within the body of the report a reprint of the very flawed and inaccurate ADA patient bulletin on the safety of dental amalgam (previously addressed in Argument 6). He also indicates that he provides copies of this ADA bulletin to patients, concerned about the mercury/amalgam controversy, who come to him for evaluation of possible mercury/amalgam hypersensitivity, and 2) Dr. Fisher references 21 scientific articles to "supposedly" support the information and positions reflected in the article. However, a careful review of the references cited left me very confused. At least 12 of the articles cited as supporting his position actually present data that is contrary to the positions expressed by Dr. Fisher.

3.   In 1975 Brun published the results of a study in which 1000 patients with contact dermatitis were tested for hypersensitivity to mercury. 11.3% of the patients tested positive to the mercury patch test. The authors also provided a comparison of their results with those published by the World Health Organization showing similar results.

4.   Nebenfuher et al. (1983) tested 1530 in-patients, 780 men and 758 women, with a routine allergy series that included mercury. Mercury allergy was found in 9.6% of those tested (91 women and 57 men).

5.   Finne et al. (1982) found that in a group of 29 patients with oral lichen planus (an inflammatory disease) 62% reacted positively to a mercury patch test. What is exciting about the Finne study is that in 4 of the patients, all of the amalgam fillings were removed and replaced by gold and composites with the following results: The lesions in 3 of these patients healed completely after an observation period of one year and in the remaining case there was a considerable improvement.

6.   Mobacken et al. (1984) reported that 16% of a group of 67 patients with oral lichen planus reacted to a mercury patch test. They found that most reactions were caused by elemental mercury.

7.   Miller et al. (1985) performed a study at Baylor College of Dentistry, Dallas, Texas involving 171 volunteer dental students (51 freshmen, 52 sophomores, 37 juniors, and 31 seniors). The authors found there was a significant correlation between the number of amalgams and the incidence of mercury hypersensitivity. One other very interesting aspect of this study was the rates of mercury hypersensitivity from freshman to seniors, which was 31%, 27%, 32%, and 39%, respectively.

It would appear from the scientific data presently available that the ADA and NIDR have grossly misrepresented the potential incidence of allergic reactions that may be directly attributable to the presence of mercury/amalgam dental fillings when they state that less than 1% of the population may be at risk. This simple statement of "less than 1%" could be the basis for tens of thousands of individuals suffering needlessly with undiagnosed conditions of mercury/amalgam hypersensitivity. I urge the ADA and the NIDR to fund the necessary research projects to determine what the "true" prevalence of mercury/amalgam allergy is in the United States.

Since publication of the original manuscript many patients and health care providers have informed me that I failed to give proper consideration to the patient who has multiple allergies to food, environmental pollutants and petrochemical based products.

If you are an individual who has diagnosed multiple allergies you require special care and treatment in the hands of a physician and dentist who are familiar and knowledgable about the mercury/amalgam relationship to your condition as well as the potential sensitivity problems that could be associated with the materials used to replace amalgams.

I am indebted to Alfred V. Zamm, M.D., F.A.C.A., F.A.C.P. of Kingston, New York who has given me permission to use some of his copyrighted patient material on this subject (Prepared with the assistance of Bruce Sorrin, D.D.S., also of Kingston, NY):

QUESTION: How can I know in advance whether removal of my mercury fillings will help me?

ANSWER: You can't. There is no way to predict this because:

1.   Allergy to mercury is not the problem in question; hence, doing skin tests to prove someone is or is not allergic to mercury is irrelevant in terms of the patient with multiple food, chemical and inhalant hypersensitivities.

2.   The patients most likely to obtain benefit are those who are most sensitive. Any lessening of any sort of the metabolic load, however small, may be significant to these ultrasensitive patients.

QUESTION: What has been the experience of other patients who have removed their mercury fillings?

ANSWER: The national data on this is limited. It is being collected via a variety of studies in the hope of determining whether a pattern exists. The following is some data I have collected that may shed some light on this new subject:

Example #1.   A patient I saw from Lake George, New York, an intelligent, high-level engineer who had been investigated by some of the outstanding clinical ecologists. This patient was a severe universal reactor. He had been unable to work, and he had been unable to eat almost all foods. He had been unable to tolerate low levels of petrochemicals. He now tolerates all of these things fairly well. Physicians were unable to help him beyond advice regarding avoidance, rotation, etc. I asked him how was he able to improve the status of his health. He told me that one physician in the Midwest told him he would not get better unless his mercury fillings (silver amalgam) were removed. He did this, and gradually his illness reversed itself (not completely).

Example #2. About six months ago one of our local H.E.A.L. (Human Ecology Action League) members decided to have the mercury fillings removed from her teeth. She was a severe universal reactor. Subsequently she sent a letter to many of us describing the reversal of her illness.

Example #3. In my own case, I felt the initiation of a benefit within two weeks after the last mercury fillings were removed (three months after the removal procedure was initiated).

Example #4. I spoke with Dr. Theron Randolph, who, as many of you know, is probably the leading authority in the country in Clinical Ecology. He told me he had suggested to about 20 patients to have the mercury fillings removed from their teeth, and that the results were mixed, i.e., there was benefit in many patients but not in everyone.

Example #5. The removal of mercury fillings is not a panacea. A patient of mine who is a universal reactor with severe ecological illness has no teeth: he wears full dentures (no fillings). His illness, therefore, must have some mechanism unrelated to mercury poisoning.

SOME FACTORS THAT MAY HELP PREDICT WHETHER A PERSON WOULD BENEFIT FROM THE REMOVAL OF THEIR MERCURY FILLINGS

To repeat, this subject is so new that this can only be taken as a supposition and conjecture:

    1) Dissimilar metals and the electrogalvanic effect.

The patient who has dissimilar metals in the mouth, i.e., one gold inlay and some mercury fillings, will have an electrogalvanic effect (a flow of electricity between these two different metals, as in a battery). The flow of electricity induces degradation of the mercury filling (silver amalgam), inducing a more rapid release of mercury than if only mercury fillings were present. This relationship will help you judge the degree to which you are at risk.

2)   Selenium.

Selenium binds with mercury to render it biologically inactive in some respects (this is why tuna is not poisoned by the mercury in its system). (Selenium is also protective against arsenic and cadmium.) One might conjecture that, if one receives some benefit from taking selenium, then the benefit may be in part due to the protective effect of selenium against mercury, hence, there might be some benefit from having the mercury fillings removed. This is not a proof, but merely conjecture.

The dose should be: One 50 microgram tablet of selenium twice a day or 1/2 dropper full twice a day of the liquid form (Dr. Zamm uses liquid selenium prepared by Nutricology Co.). Some patients who are petrochemically sensitive become tolerant to petrochemical exposure on this dose.

Petrochemically sensitive patients sometimes react to very small quantities of selenium. For the very sensitive, the initiation of selenium should be under the guidance of a physician who is knowledgeable in this subject.

When benefit ensues, some patients note a benefit within a few days; in others, it may take up to three months to notice a benefit.

3)   Zinc.

Mercury competes biologically with zinc and is in the same column of the periodic table. Some patients experience some improvement of their general well-being with zinc. The possible reasons are multiple. One reason might be the relationship described above, i.e., zinc is protective to some extent against mercury. Although this too is no proof but merely conjecture, it is something to think about in terms of trying to portend a benefit from the removal of one's mercury fillings.

The dose of zinc is one 15 milligram tablet once a day. Too much can also present problems. More is not necessarily better.

When benefit ensues, it may be apparent within a day or two.

4)   Thiamine (Vitamin B1).

Take thiamine (vitamin B1) 50 milligrams with breakfast and 50 milligrams with supper. Look for significant benefit, i.e, greater energy, greater well-being, etc. If it's going to work, the benefits will generally be noted within 6-12 hours after taking the first dose and certainly by the next morning. If benefit results, this benefit could be considered an additional piece of evidence in favor of suspecting that mercury might be acting as a poison. Remember: at this stage of our knowledge about dental mercury, this is no proof but merely conjecture. It is something to think about, however, in terms of trying to predict if a benefit will ensue from the removal of one's mercury dental fillings.

HOW CAN MY DENTIST WORK ON ME AND MINIMIZE MY PROVOCATION? WHAT TO DO BEFORE, DURING AND AFTER THE DENTAL PROCEDURE?

ANSWER: Your dentist must be sympathetic to the idea that a person could be hypersensitive to the degree with which we are all familiar. Polite lip service is insufficient. Many dentists, physicians, and other health care professionals simply do not have the personal experience with such hypersensitive people and find it hard to appreciate the subtleties necessary to deal with such people.

Hence, written instructions (typed preferred) should be given to your dentist prior to starting this procedure. The patient should be satisfied that there is a sympathetic and understanding person knowledgeable in chemical hypersensitivity at the other end of the drill.

The above information taken from Dr. Zamm's patient literature is primarily oriented towards the patient with multiple allergies. Dr. Zamm goes into much greater detail in advising his patients how to prepare for dental treatment. He also provides a set of guidelines for the dentist treating patients with multiple allergies, outlining the special considerations that may be necessary during treatment.

The patient with known and diagnosed allergies has a responsibility to insure that the dentist has been made aware of this fact prior to commencement of any dental procedures.

NOTE: Patients or dentists desiring a copy of Dr. Zamm's booklet, please send $2.00 and a self-addressed stamped envelope to Dr. Alfred V. Zamm, 111 Maiden Lane, Kingston, NY 12401.

REFERENCES

1. Djerassi E. and Berova N. The possibilities of allergic reaction from silver amalgam restorations. International Dental Journal, Vol. 19, No. 4:481-488, 1969.

2. Rudner et al. Epidemiology of contact dermatitis in North America: 1972. Archives of Dermatology, Vol. 108, No. 4:537-540, 1973.

3. Brun R. Epidemiology of contact dermatitis in Geneva (1000 cases). Contact Dermatitis, Vol. 1:214-217, 1975.

4. Fisher A.A. The misuse of the patch test to determine "hypersensitivity" to mercury amalgam dental fillings. CUTIS, Vol. 35, No. 2:110-117, 1985.

5. Nebenfuhrer L. et al. Mercury allergy in Budapest. Contact Dermatitis, Vol. 10, No. 2:121-122, 1983.

6. Finne K. et al. Oral lichen planus and contact allergy to mercury. International Journal of Oral Surgery, Vol. 11:236-239, 1982.

7. Mobacken et al. Oral lichen planus: Hypersensitivity to dental restoration material. Contact Dermatitis, Vol. 10:11-15, 1984.

8. Miller E.G. et al. Prevalence of mercury hypersensitivity in dental students. Journal of Dental Research, Vol. 64, Special Issue, Page 338, Abstract #1472, March, 1985.

9. Zamm A.V. Mercury and Dentistry. Patient literature, 1985. Kingston New York.

CHAPTER 13

POSTERIOR COMPOSITE DENTAL FILLING MATERIALS

Much has happened in this area since the original manuscript for the book was written. The use of the new composite materials for posterior dental restorations has literally exploded and although they have not given full approval, the ADA has given provisional approval to three different brand name posterior composites.

Dr. Karl Leinfelder, one of the foremost researchers and authorities on composite materials stated during a scientific presentation at the 1984 ADA Annual meeting in Atlanta: "From 1981 to 1983, amalgam moved from having 72% of the market to having 49%; composites moved from 28% to 51%. I expect this trend will continue in 1984."

I would have to conclude from Dr. Leinfelder's remarks that a great number of practicing dentists are using composite materials in lieu of amalgam. I also feel certain that many of these dentists are aware of the "mercury" problem and would seriously consider converting their practices to mercury-free if the ADA would only modify their public position concerning the unquestioned safety of amalgam as a dental material.

The ADA has publicly stated that the average amalgam restoration last 10 years. However, the validity of the 10 year figure is questionable. In a study by Hamilton et al. (1983) only 17% of the original amalgam fillings in molars were still functional at the end of 10 years. In another study by Maryniuk (1984) titled "In Search of Treatment Longevity — a 30 Year Perspective" the author concluded after reviewing all available literature on the subject that the average lifespan of an amalgam filling appeared to be 5.5 to 11.5 years.

I raise the point of longevity because the ADA has made an issue of it. One of their positions appears to be that amalgam restorations last an average of 10 years, whereas it is not known how long composites will last. The last part of the sentence is true. Longevity studies of posterior composites are incomplete at this point in time because of their newness. However, there have been several studies of two or more years duration that indicate favorable wear characteristics. Moreover, longevity is not the real issue in this controversy. The real issue is material toxicity. There is adequate acceptable scientific data to bring the biocompatibility of mercury/amalgam into serious question. Conversely, a literature review of available scientific data indicates that composite materials are reasonably biocompatible and do not have harmful characteristics when placed properly.

The last statement made above is extremely important. *The proper placement of posterior composite materials is critically technique sensitive.* The dentist must know the proper base material to use in covering the exposed dentin, the correct protocols for placing the base material, the correct acid etching technique, the correct cement or bonding agent to use and the correct equipment and protocols for placing and curing the composite material. In each of these areas I do not believe the ADA has provided the leadership needed. As a result, until recently, those dentists using these materials have had to arrive at the proper protocols and materials through trial and error and the exchange of information with their colleagues. That is not the situation today as there has been a proliferation of books, video courses and seminars on the proper placement of composites.

Another aspect of placing posterior composites that you should be aware of is that the proper placement of a composite restoration is much more time consuming in comparison to amalgam. Consequently, your dentist will have to charge more than he would for an amalgam. A recent study by Dilley et al (1985) showed that composite restorations required 35 percent longer to place than a similar amalgam filling. The net result to the patient is a higher unit cost per surface for composite restorations versus amalgam fillings.

One problem that appeared early on with the use of the new composites was that of post operative pain and thermal sensitivity (reaction to hot or cold). Subsequent research and patient experience has indicated that this phenomenon was primarily related to some of the earlier bases and cements that were being placed in direct contact with the dentin to seal it.

The newer materials and information on proper placement techniques available today have dramatically reduced the post operative problems. The use of glass ionomer base material and certain other cements properly applied have proven effective in totally sealing the dentin and pulp resulting in minimal or no irritation at all to these tissues. With the dentin and pulp properly protected the phenomenon of pain and thermal sensitivity have been effectively controlled for most individuals. Bear in mind that the trauma caused during any operative procedure, regardless of the material being used, can also cause post operative pain and thermal sensitivity.

Some people however may still experience an initial sensitivity to hot or cold that will dissipate over time. During this period your dentist may recommend the use of certain desensitizing tooth pastes. However, if the pain or sensitivity persists you should advise your dentist. This is true for any dental procedure regardless of the type of material that was placed in your mouth i.e., gold, composite, etc. We are all biochemically individual which means that you could possibly react to something that normally doesn't cause any problems in other people. Remember, your dentist can't help you if he doesn't know a problem exists.

A major advantage concerning the use of composite is that much less of your natural tooth structure is lost in preparing the tooth for reconstruction. That is because the materials are all bonded together with the remaining natural tooth structure and results indicate the actual restoration of the tooth to 98% of its predecayed state. The preparation for the placement of an amalgam filling is much different because much more of the natural tooth structure must be cut away in order to provide for mechanical retention of the amalgam once it is condensed into the cavity. Amalgam doesn't restore or bond to anything in the natural tooth structure and achieves its seal only through mechanical condensation.

In this regard it is interesting to note that Dr. Harold Loe, Director of the National Institute of Dental Research, appeared on the March 13, 1985 ABC Good Morning America Show and, in essence, stated the following, Composites bind to the tooth and you get a good restoration. What is happening now is that these materials are being used in posterior teeth and this means we can get rid of gold and silver. The composites are synthetic materials that are very attractive from a cosmetic point of view—but they also stick to the tooth substance, so a major portion of the drilling that has been used in the past to prepare cavities to retain silver and gold is going to be reduced dramatically.

It would appear from Dr. Loe's statement on national television that the National Institute of Dental Research has embraced the use of composites in posterior teeth. That and the fact that the ADA has provisionally approved three different posterior composite materials should dictate that all dental insurance plans provide full payment for composite fillings rather than pay only what their rate schedule allows for amalgam fillings.

A frequent and serious concern of patients contemplating having their amalgams replaced with composite restorations usually centers around two questions: 1) Is replacing amalgams dangerous? and 2) Is it true that I must have the amalgams replaced in a very specific sequence based on their electrical readings?

IS REPLACING AMALGAMS DANGEROUS?

As indicated previously, aside from the possibility that a composite restoration may not last as long as an amalgam filling, (bear in mind that only time will prove that statement) the biocompatibility of the new composite materials is really not an issue.

The ADA has made the following policy statement on this subject: "The Association wishes to emphasize that, except in individuals sensitive to mercury, there is no reason why a patient should seek at this time to have amalgam restorations (silver fillings) removed. Indeed, the effect of such a procedure and further restorative operations could be detrimental to the patient's oral health, including the unnecessary loss of teeth, and cannot be justified."

What is wrong about the ADA statement is that it doesn't present the true picture and is actually a disservice to the patient and the dentist. The facts of the matter are:

(1) Dentists routinely remove amalgam fillings every day and replace them with another amalgam filling. It appears that the ADA is saying that it is just not acceptable to replace amalgam with any other dental material. In reality, there is no basis for the ADA position.

(2) Most amalgam fillings are replaced because of decay under the filling, excessive corrosion, fracture, etc. The procedure is so commonplace, that insurance companies will pay for replacement of an amalgam filling after only one year.

(3) Certainly, there are situations that are beyond the control of your dentist which may cause you to lose a tooth. However, the newer materials are so much more flexible and advantageous to work with that in many instances, teeth can be saved that would otherwise be lost if amalgam was the only material available.

A major concern of most patients is the question of how much mercury vapor they may be exposed to by having their amalgams replaced. *There are special techniques that should be utilized by your dentist to remove amalgam fillings.* If done properly, there is a minimum exposure to the release of mercury vapor caused by the removal procedure. However, as a patient there are certain aspects related to removal of amalgams that you should be aware of:

(1) The office and operatory should be well ventilated.

(2) The dentist should have an assistant present to assist in minimizing their exposure and yours to any mercury vapor. The correct protocol requires the use of high volumes of cold water both from the drill and separate irrigation by the assistant who should also simultaneously be using high volume suction to evacuate the vapor and particles resulting from the removal procedure.

(3) In some dental offices the dentist may ask you to breathe through a nose piece that will permit you to draw air from another

area of the operatory. Or, if the dentist has nitrous oxide available and you have elected to use it, this will accomplish the same thing.

(4) During the procedure, the dentist and assistant are at greater risk for exposure to mercury vapor than the patient. So, don't be surprised if you see them put on special masks and surgical gloves as these are necessary to protect them during repeated removal operations.

DO I HAVE TO HAVE MY AMALGAMS REMOVED IN A SPECIAL SEQUENCE?

There is no scientific documentation to support the idea that sequential removal is essential to achieving any benefits from amalgam replacement. The subject has been investigated by some highly respected scientists and no basis can be found.

Dentists all over the world routinely replace amalgam fillings with nonmetal restorations without any regard to the specific sequence of removal. In this country, dentists who have switched from sequential removal based on electrical evaluation, to removal or replacement without any regard to electrical current, have stated that have noticed no difference in benefits that accrue to their patients.

These facts not withstanding, if your dentist wishes to remove and replace your amalgam fillings sequentially, there is absolutely nothing wrong in doing it that way.

REFERENCES

1. Leinfelder K.F. Presentation made during the Scientific Session of the ADA annual meeting, October 1984, Atlanta, GA and reported in the Journal of the American Dental Association, Vol. 109, No. 6:893, 1984.

2. Hamilton et al. Marginal fracture not a predictor of longevity for two dental amalgam alloys: A ten-year study. Journal of Prosthetic Dentistry, Vol. 50, No. 2:200-202, 1983.

3. Maryniuk G.A. In search of treatment longevity—a 30 year perspective. Journal of the American Dental Association, Vol. 109, No. 5:739-744, 1984.

4. The Posterior Composite Reporter, Volumes 1 and 2, 1985. Maxplax Ltd., Mississauga, Ontario, Canada.

5. Dilley D.H. et al. Time required for placement of alloy versus resin posterior restorations. Journal of Dental Research, Vol. 64, Special Issue, Page 340, Abstract #1583, March, 1985.

Chapter 14
WHAT CAN I DO?

The first thing that you must do, is make an individual and personal decision about what you have read. If you do not believe that the mercury in dental amalgam or dissimilar metals in the mouth represent a potentially serious health hazard, then merely count the time expended reading this book as "contributing to your total store of interesting facts" and turn your attention to other things.

If, on the other hand, you reach a conclusion that there appears to be some basis to the statements that dissimilar metals can create electrical havoc in your body and that mercury and other metals escaping from dental amalgam and entering your body constitute potentially serious threats to human health then, be assured, there are a whole range of actions that you can take. On the personal level, here are some of the actions you can take:

1. This action involves the simple act of requesting that your elected representatives and the appropriate agencies of the federal government resolve the questions. Suitable research projects and protocols must be established and funded to answer the questions scientifically.

A. Write to the Chairman of the Subcommittee on Health and Safety, United States Congress. Call your local Congressional representatives office to get the correct name and address of to whom you should address your letter.

(1) Express your personal concerns regarding the safety of mercury amalgam dental fillings.

(2) If you have had your mercury amalgam dental fillings replaced with resultant improvement of your health, send a brief case history outlining the facts.

(3) In 1984 the National Institute of Dental Research

(NIDR) recommended that research studies be initiated to determine the biocompatibility and safety of dental amalgam. In 1994, ten years later, the NIDR has not funded adequate research to scientifically resolve the amalgam controversy. Request an answer as to why the National Institute of Dental Research has not funded appropriate research projects investigating the biocompatibility and safety of mercury amalgam as a dental material.

(4) Demand to know how it is possible that the Food and Drug Administration has permitted the dental profession to routinely implant a poisonous material in your body without complying with any of the standards and controls established for other implant materials used by the medical profession.

(5) Demand to know how it is possible for the dental profession to implant a poison in your body without the need to advise you that it is doing so, or obtain your consent to do so.

B. Write to the Director, National Institutes of Health, 14 North Drive, Bethesda, MD 20814.

Request that you be provided with the scientific proof supporting statements made by the various divisions under the Director's control, and the ADA, that the mercury escaping from dental amalgams and being absorbed by the body causes no pathological damage and does not constitute a health hazard. Specify that you do not want opinions resulting from meetings and conferences but, hard scientific research findings supporting the safety of amalgam.

Ask how it is possible that in all the billions of dollars expended on research projects, nobody has ever demanded that toxicological research on heavy metals include dental mercury amalgam as a source.

2. One thing you can do easily in the comfort of your own home is to play detective on yourself. Take a sheet of paper and start jotting down the approximate dates of when your chronic or persistent symptoms of health problems started

appearing. For example, when you first started feeling extremely tired or fatigued all the time, or when you first started having a severe acne, or when did you first notice that metallic taste in your mouth, etc. In this regard, you might consult the Chapter 8 listing of symptoms and pick out the ones you have and note when they started.

Next, to the best of your knowledge, jot down the dates when you first had any dental restoration work done, and all subsequent dates when additional work was done. Remember now, we are also talking about dissimilar metals and this would include the installation of any metal in your mouth, including orthodontic devices.

Lastly, line up the two sets of dates and see if there is any relationship between when you first experienced the symptoms and when you had the dental work done. You might turn up some astonishing correlations.

3. If you have been under a physician's care for any of the diseases or syndrome type health conditions (collections of symptoms) for which there is no established etiology or cause and you have mercury amalgam dental fillings in your mouth then you should consider taking some of the following action:

Return to your physician and discuss with him the possibility that mercury hypersensitivity or intoxication may be involved. If he or she doesn't think much of the idea, then start calling other physicians until you find one who has an open mind, has knowledge on the subjects of mercury toxicity and/or hypersensitivity, and is willing to work with you to try and find an answer. (At the end of this chapter there is a list of medical, dental and other organizations that may be able to assist you in finding a health professional sympathetic to your needs.)

An Allergist or Clinical Ecologist may be able to determine if you are hypersensitive to mercury, or some of the other metals contained in the amalgam. However, as indicated previously in the book, there is quite a bit of controversy concerning the patch test. This includes: Disagreement over what is the right material to use for testing - i.e., mercuric chloride or ammoniated mercury, the correct dilution - i.e., 1% or 2% or 5%; and is the determination of a positive reaction based only on a dermatological reaction on the skin under the patch or are there possible systemic reactions? Further, if you are already sensitized to mercury, the application of a mercury patch to your skin may aggravate your sensitivity. Moreover, there is some confusion over interpretation of the results of the test. These facts notwithstanding, in the hands of a skilled clinician who has had experience with mercury, you may be able to obtain diagnostic information that will be important to your final decision.

NOTE: It is highly questionable whether a mercury patch test should, under any circumstances, ever be give to pregnant women, diagnosed cases of Systemic Lupus Erythematosus, Multiple Sclerosis, Leukemia, Hodgkins disease, cardiovascular disease, mental illness (especially manic depression), Acrodynia, and MLNS (Kawasaki's disease). If you have made up your mind to have your mercury amalgam fillings replaced, do not take the mercury patch test.

There are some other ways available to you and your health care provider to determine whether your mercury amalgam fillings and/or dissimilar metals are contributing to your total body burden of mercury or generating electrogalvanic action at levels that may have the potential to cause some problems.

(1) The Jerome Mercury Vapor Analyzer may be used to determine intra-oral mercury vapor levels. This is a simple non-invasive test to record how much mercury vapor is being released from your mercury amalgam fillings when stimulated. Readings are taken in your mouth before and after chewing gum for 10 minutes. High readings would tend to confirm that your dental fillings are releasing mercury vapor whenever they are stimulated by chewing, drinking hot

fluids, brushing your teeth, etc., and that you are inhaling this mercury vapor, thereby contributing to your total body burden of mercury. NOTE: This is not a diagnostic test for mercury toxicity. Consequently, it can only provide information demonstrating that there is mercury vapor being released intra-orally and inhaled. Hopefully, in the not too distant future, there may be computer simulation models available that may have diagnostic capabilities. These will utilize the recorded intra-oral mercury vapor readings together with the numbers and surfaces of mercury amalgam fillings in your mouth to calculate the contribution to total mercury body burden, as well as provide data on what the accumulation in various organs and tissues may be. This data would then become part of a risk-assessment evaluation.

(2) Your dentist may have a device sensitive enough to measure electrogalvanic currents or electrical potentials. If so, he may be able to demonstrate whether or not the dissimilar metals in your mouth are creating an electrogalvanic environment. High readings could possibly be involved in a number of problems such as unexplained pain, headaches, or even temporomandibular join (TMJ) dysfunction in addition to causing increased corrosion and increased release of mercury and other ions from dental alloys. Remember, this is only a demonstration that electrogalvanic currents are present. It is not a diagnosis of mercury toxicity or hypersensitivity. Nor can current readings (with an ammeter) be used to compare one filling to another in the oral cavity.

(3) Traditionally, simple periodontal disease (periodontitis) has been related to a variety of local irritants, such as subgingival plaque formation, the presence of certain bacteria, impaction of food, and rough edges of fillings. However, the textbooks and scientific literature establish that mercury and/or amalgam fillings can pathologically damage periodontal tissue. Further, some of the symptoms shown in Chapter 8 under "Oral Cavity Disorders" are considered

classical symptoms of mercury toxicity. Consequently, if you have periodontal problems it may be another factor that your dentist or physician should consider in attempting to determine if mercury amalgam fillings are a causative factor in your health problems.

(4) Hair analysis. Although subject to contamination from hair care products that may contain mercury and atmospheric mercury, a hair analysis reflecting high levels of mercury would be an additional indication that mercury should be considered in the diagnostic process.

(5) Urine mercury levels. Although unreliable in determining chronic exposures to low levels of mercury, this may provide usable diagnostic information. You may also wish to have urine selenium levels determined at the same time, as there is scientific evidence that mercury causes increased excretion of selenium. Low or normal levels of urine mercury in the presence of high urine selenium levels might warrant additional consideration regarding the true status of your mercury body burden.

(6) The same thing can be stated for mercury levels in the blood. Unfortunately, the results provide very inconclusive correlations to tissue toxicity. There is some information in the scientific literature indicating that mercury content of red blood cells is a better indicator.

(7) There is a great deal of interest and research in progress related to total White Blood Cell and T-cell and B-cell lymphocyte counts. These indices are all involved with the status of the immune system and there is preliminary evidence indicating changes in T-cell B-cell differentials (the ratio of T cell count to the B cell count) may be related to the presence of mercury amalgam and/or nickel. If the tests show decreased values that can't be attributed to other causes, it should suggest to your physician that serious consideration be given to the possibility that mercury amalgam fillings may be the causative factor.

Your physician may wish to utilize a diagnostic chelation challenge protocol, using drugs or amino acids that have been shown to complex or bind with mercury. Urinalysis while undergoing this type of protocol will indicate whether you are excreting increased amounts of mercury in your urine. This could provide an indication of an excessive total body burden of mercury. There may also be an amelioration of some symptoms. Both of these results would be additional factors implicating mercury.

If your particular philosophy of life does not encompass the taking of drugs, the detoxification of mercury may also be accomplished to some degree with certain vitamins, minerals, and amino acids. The information that follows has been taken from the scientific literature and each nutrient mentioned has been shown to be biochemically involved in either assisting the body to eliminate mercury or in reducing the metabolic damage mercury can cause.

Scientific research has demonstrated that mercury has a great affinity for the sulfur molecule. The primary sulfur-containing amino acids are cysteine, methionine and taurine. Whenever mercury attaches or binds to the sulfur-containing molecules in these amino acids, it reduces their availability for normal metabolic functions. Consequently, the principle behind increasing your intake of sulfur-containing amino acids is to 1) provide additional binding sites for the mercury and 2) insure there is an adequate supply to accomplish normal biochemical functions. Sulfur containing compounds of biochemical importance include insulin, prolactin, growth hormone and vasopressin. Cysteine, along with pantothenic acid, is a precursor of coenzyme A.

CYSTEINE

Cysteine is very soluble in water and therefore can be easily eliminated via the urine. However, cysteine can become oxidized to cystine, which can then present the potential of forming kidney stones. Research has demonstrated that if an adequate supply of vitamin C is available, it will keep the cysteine in its reduced and soluble form, thereby preventing the formation of stones. The ratio of vitamin C to cysteine is three to one. Cysteine reacts readily with many substances and recent research indicates that there may be some problems with supplementing cysteine. Therefore, until further scientific research clarifies the situation, you should not supplement with cysteine, but rather insure that your diet provides adequately for your cysteine requirements. Your body can produce cysteine from methionine. Therefore, if you want to supplement, do so with methionine.

METHIONINE

Methionine is one of the essential amino acids required by humans, whereas cysteine is considered to be nonessential. Methionine is the precursor for the manufacture of cysteine in the body, so extra supplementation of this critical amino acid should increase available cysteine. Low concentrations of mercury have been shown to inhibit methionine uptake by a factor of 2.

TAURINE

Taurine is a sulfur-containing amino acid that the body makes from cysteine. Methionine is a precursor for cysteine and taurine biosynthesis. Taurocholic acid is one of two bile acids needed to break down fats. Your body cannot produce taurocholic acid unless an adequate supply of Taurine is available. Scientists have also determined that taurine plays a major role in controlling the transport of blood electrolytes such as calcium and potassium and, because of this, may play an important role in the heart and cardiovascular system.

GLUTATHIONE

Glutathione is a sulfur-containing tripeptide composed of glutamic acid, cysteine and glycine. Glutathione is present in almost all cells in rather high concentrations and serves as a reservoir and transport form of cysteine. The cysteine component of glutathione is protected from conversion to the insoluble cystine. Because of this quality, there is some research indicating glutathione to be preferable to cysteine when supplementing in a detoxification protocol. Glutathione can also replace cysteine derived from methionine, thus exerting a methionine sparing action, which will be of benefit when supplementing with both glutathione and methionine.

Glutathione has a biological role in the antioxidant recycling process. Both vitamin C and E require the presence of an adequate supply of reduced glutathione for regeneration from their oxidized and inactivated state after participating in the free radical scavenger process. Glutathione also plays a role in the effectiveness of selenium.

VITAMIN C

Some of the physiological functions of vitamin C in the body are: absorption of iron from the gut; maintenance of the adrenal cortex; wound healing; formation of cartilage, dentine, bone and teeth; metabolism of tryptophan, phenylalanine, and tyrosine; synthesis of collagen; maintenance of capillaries; growth; chelating agent for heavy metals and a major role as an antioxidant.

It is the last two functions that are involved in the detoxification process. Research has demonstrated that mercury is able to generate or cause an increase in free radicals. The nutrients considered to have an antioxidant function in the body are so designated because of their involvement in suppressing or controlling free radical generation.

Blackstone, 1974, using guinea-pigs, demonstrated that mercury significantly reduced the concentration of ascorbic acid in the brain, adrenals and spleen of animals receiving maintenance doses of the vitamin.

Vitamin C works synergistically with vitamin E. This means that the functions of vitamin E are enhanced when there is an adequate supply of ascorbic acid present. Stated another way, vitamin C acts to reduce the rate of oxidative consumption of vitamin E.

VITAMIN E

The scientific literature shows that vitamin E can reduce the toxic effects of mercury. There is also evidence that vitamin E protects vitamin A during digestion and absorption and also when both are present in tissues.

Fukine et al., (1984) demonstrated lipid peroxidation and a decrease in vitamin E content in the rat kidney 12 hours after mercury administration. Laboratory test by other researchers have demonstrated that vitamin E was able to reduce the chromosomal breakage caused by mercury.

SELENIUM

It is paradoxical that although selenium can be toxic by itself it also prevents the toxicity of several heavy metals such as silver, mercury, cadmium and lead (Forst 1972). There are many studies showing that selenium has been able to reduce the toxicity of mercury. However, the exact means by which this is accomplished is still not clear. One theory involves the fact that selenium as an essential constituent of glutathione peroxidase, which is an enzyme that metabolically possesses the ability to destroy hydrogen peroxide and organic hydroperoxides. If mercury is capable of generating peroxides as an oxidation by-product, then the role of selenium in controlling these peroxide radicals seems plausible. Another possible mechanism would be that selenium closely resembles sulfur in its physical and chemical properties. The latter role may be the reason selenium is effective in binding mercury. Mercury's strongest affinity is for selenium

Autopsy studies done by Kosta, Byrne and Zelenko in 1975 revealed that, contrary to accepted belief that the kidney was the prime accumulator of inorganic mercury, the thyroid and pituitary had retained and accumulated more inorganic mercury than the kidney. They also found that an approximate 1.1 molar ratio, selenium to mercury, existed for those organs that accumulated and retained mercury strongly. This type of ratio suggested a direct mercury-selenium linkage and the authors concluded that the co-accumulation of selenium with mercury may be a natural or auto-protective effect.

ZINC

Zinc is an essential component of approximately 100 different enzymes. Although our knowledge is limited, at present there is evidence that mercury will inhibit the following zinc-involved enzymes or coenzymes: alcohol dehydrogenase; delta-aminolevulinic acid dehydrogenase; carbonic anhydrase; alkaline phosphatase and aldolase. The hormone insulin is stored as a zinc complex and, although I was not able to find research indicating that mercury affects the function of insulin, I was able to find some biochemical pathways where it might well be involved. This might explain why some anecdotal case histories reflect amelioration or clearing of some blood sugar problems when the mercury body burden is reduced.

Zinc is involved in the synthesis of a low weight protein in the body called metallothionein. I suppose a simplified definition would be 'a protein that contains one or more specific metals in addition to amino acids.' It is also a protein that has an affinity for some of the heavy metals. Experiments with rats done by Day, Funk and Brady in 1984 demonstrated that mercury could displace zinc from metallothionein. Their study, as well as many others, considers zinc-induced synthesis of metallothionein as perhaps the primary factor in reducing the toxicity of many heavy metals. One other important reason for the inclusion of zinc in any detoxification protocol is that there is evidence showing that cysteine can cause the increased excretion of zinc. Therefore, in any effort to reduce the body burden of mercury or reduce it's toxic effects, it appears prudent to insure that there is an adequate intake of zinc.

Zinc works synergistically with vitamin B6 and Vitamin E. Also, vitamin B6 increases zinc absorption significantly.

VITAMIN B1 (Thiamine)

Vitamin B1 also contains a sulfur group and has been used (50-100 mg as an intramuscular injection) to treat mercury poisoning. The vitamin has a rapid turnover in the brain and heart and the levels are reduced by mercury exposure (mercury oxidizes thiamine to thiochrome).(See Moeschlin S.).   Ziff has demonstrated that the symptoms of B1 deficiency and mercury poisoning are almost identical. Further, recent research revealed by Hendler has shown that a thiamine deficiency can result in disturbed heart rhythm, shortness of breath, swelling of the feet and legs, low blood pressure, chest and abdominal pain, kidney failure, cardiac failure and, if not corrected, death. Unfortunately, medical scientists are not as yet evaluating or correlating mercury body burden as a possible etiological factor in heart disease.

VITAMIN B6

Vitamin B6 is involved in the manner in which the body handles the transfer of sulfur. There is also evidence that B6 functions as a coenzyme of the enzyme responsible for the synthesis of cystathione from homocysteine and serine and a cleavage enzyme responsible for the conversion of cystathionine to cysteine. This whole cascade of biochemical events is involved in the metabolism of methionine. So here again is another major biochemical pathway for sulfur, in which B6 is intimately involved. Mercury's great affinity for the sulfur molecule would indicate that B6 is also involved in how the body handles the detoxification of mercury. There is also evidence that a deficiency of vitamin B6 is accompanied by an impairment of the immune system.

CALCIUM PANTOTHENATE OR PANTOTHENIC ACID

This vitamin, also known as vitamin B5, is a major constituent of the adrenal glands and as such may be involved in how your body handles stress. In regard to the adrenal glands, vitamin C is also stored in the adrenals and is rapidly depleted under stress conditions.

The physiological active form of pantothenic acid is coenzyme A and as such, serves as a cofactor for a variety of enzymatic actions and hormonal actions in the body. There is scientific evidence that mercury can inhibit or suppress coenzyme A. It is interesting to note that coenzyme A is also a cofactor involved in the synthesis of steroid hormones (adrenal function). Here again cysteine is involved in the biochemical process, reacting with a derivative of pantothenic acid to form coenzyme A.

ACIDOPHILUS

A recent article by Rowland et al. (1984) demonstrated that the intestinal microflora may play a significant role in determining the excretion rate of mercury: "Treatment of mice with antibiotics throughout the experimental period to suppress the gut flora reduced fecal mercury excretion and the dietary differences in whole body retention of mercury." A logical extension of this research to humans undergoing any detoxification protocol would be to insure that intestinal microflora are not suppressed. Acidophilus, yogurt (unsweetened and with active culture) or buttermilk are considered beneficial in restoring intestinal microflora.

It is apparent as we progress through the nutrients that are involved in the detoxification process, that most appear to have some relationship to each other - i.e., vitamin C protects cysteine from conversion to cystine and reduces the oxidation of vitamin E; glutathione not only functions as a storage and carrier vehicle for cysteine but is involved in the clinical effectiveness of vitamin C, E, and selenium; vitamin E protects vitamin A, and functions more effectively in the presence of vitamin C, glutathione and selenium; zinc works synergistically with vitamin B6 and E; vitamin B6 enhances the absorption of zinc and is critical in transporting sulfur and the metabolic conversion of methionine to cysteine; pantothenic acid is the active form of coenzyme A and as such is involved in many biochemical processes which involve many of the other nutrients mentioned; and acidophilus appears to be essential to the health of the gut micro flora, which not only are involved in the assimilation of nutrients ingested but are also critical to the elimination of some forms of mercury from the body.

It should be readily apparent that the proper way of utilizing this information is under the care of a physician, dentist or other health professional who has studied the complex field of Nutrition. It is also essential that whoever is supervising your care should have taken the time and effort to become thoroughly informed on the subject of mercury toxicity and it's relationship to mercury amalgam dental fillings.

For those of you who are adamant about self-care, there are many nutritional products available (at most health food stores) that have been formulated specifically to assist in the detoxification of free radicals and heavy metals. Unless you have read extensively on nutrition and have a fundamental understanding of the biochemical functions of the body, these pre-formulated products will be simpler to take and may be just as effective as taking the individual nutrients. If you wish to increase your intake of a particular component of the formula, you can easily do so by supplementing those nutrients separately.

It should be obvious from the information provided in this chapter that there is a critical need for definitive laboratory tests to allow the physician to make a differential diagnosis of mercury toxicity. Hopefully research funds will be allocated by the responsible government agencies to accomplish this. In the mean time you must understand that there is no single test that will tell you categorically that amalgams and/or electrogalvanic potentials are the cause of your problems. In many cases it will be a subjective judgement similar to concluding "that where there's smoke, there could be fire."

You personally have to be the ultimate judge of how much proof you need in order to make up your own mind that the health problems you have been experiencing may be related to your amalgam fillings or dissimilar metals in your mouth. If you decide that there is a very probable relationship and you want to proceed with removal of the metals and replacement with the new composites, exercise caution. A great number of dentist are still not familiar with the new composite materials used for posterior restorations or the proper techniques for their correct placement.

Don't be bashful. Ask your dentist which brand(s) of composites he has been using and how long he has been using them. Ask if the manufacturer has stated that the material is acceptable for posterior use and whether they have provided at least a two year scientific study proving the claims they make. Have your dentist explain exactly what the recommended treatment plan is going to be and what you can expect to happen.

In most instances, use of detoxification nutrients and the removal of the amalgam fillings will cause a redistribution of mercury within your body. This fact, together with the possibility of a temporary increase in mercury body burden resulting from the amalgam removal process, may cause an exacerbation of your symptoms. Your dentist should be completely familiar with the nutritional support/detoxification protocol that you should be on concurrently with any removal of amalgams, and the length of time you should remain on such protocols. Where a great number of amalgam surfaces are involved, your dentist should schedule you for multiple appointments. A prudent approach would be no more than one quadrant a month, giving your body a chance to adjust and compensate prior to the next appointment.

Replacement of your mercury amalgam fillings with nonmetal or gold is no panacea. Some individuals may begin to experience relief or amelioration of symptomatology within the first week after some of the amalgams have been replaced. Others may not experience any changes until all of the amalgams have been replaced and their body has had sufficient time to excrete and reduce the total body burden of mercury. This can take anywhere from one week to more than a year after the last amalgam has been removed, dependent on your own biochemical status.

Finally, there are those of you who may not experience any relief or changes in symptomatology. Remember, each of us has a specific biochemical individuality that will ultimately determine how we respond. No matter what the outcome, you will have done one thing that is irrefutable. You will have eliminated an implanted poison from your body and in those individuals where dissimilar metals can be totally eliminated, you will have removed the source for the generation of any potentially harmful electrical currents.

Following are the names and addresses of some organizations that may be able to assist you in finding a physician, dentist or other health professional familiar with the problems outline in this book;

- Foundation For Toxic Free Dentistry, P.O. Box 608010, Orlando, FL 32860-8010.

- International Academy of Oral Medicine and Toxicology. P.O. Box P.O. Box 608531, Orlando, FL 32860-8531.

- American College of Advancement in Medicine 23121 Verbugo Dr., Suite 204; Laguna Hills, CA 92653 714-583-7666.

- American Academy of Biological Dentistry P.O. Box 856; Carmel Valley, CA 93924.

- American Academy of Environmental Medicine, P.O. Box 16106, Denver, CO 80216.

- American Holistic Medical Association 4101 Lake Boone Trail, Suite 201 Raleigh, NC 27607.

- Environmental Dental Association. 9974 Scripps Ranch Blvd., Suite #36, San Diego, CA 92131.

- Holistic Dental Association, Inc. 974 North 21st St., Newark, OH 43055.

- Huggins Diagnostic Center. 5080 List Dr., Colorado Springs, CO 80919.

- Queen and Company Health Communications, Inc. P.O. Box 49308; Colorado Springs, CO 80819-9938.

- Dr. Jerry Mittleman 263 West End Ave., #2A; New York, NY 10023.

- National Center for Homeopathy 801 North Fairfax St., Suite 306 Alexandria, VA 22314.

REFERENCES

Bilbert M.M. and Specher J. Protective effect of vitamin E on genotoxicity of methyl mercury. J of Toxicol and Environ Health, Vol. 12:767-773, 1983.

Binkley F. et al. Pyridoxine and the transfer of sulfur. J Biol Chem. Vol. 194:109-113, 1952.

Blackstone S. et al. Some interrelationships between vitamin C (L ascorbic acid) and mercury in the guinea-pig. Food Cosmet Toxicol, Vol. 12:511-516, 1974.

Chang A.-S. and Maines M.D. Effect of selenium on glutathione metabolism. Induction of y-glutamylcysteine synthetase and glutathione reductase in the rat liver. Biochem Pharmacol. Vol. 30 No. 23:3217-3223, 1981.

Day F.A. et al. In vivo and ex vivo displacement of zinc from metallothionein by cadmium and by mercury. Chem Biol Interactions, Vol. 50, No. 2:159-174, 1984.

Eftychis H. and Anderson R. Prevention of induction of suppressor activity in human mononuclear leukocytes by ascorbate and cysteine. Int. J. Vitamin Nutrition Research, Vol. 53, No.4:398-401, 1983.

Fukino H. et al. Effect of zinc pretreatment on mercuric chloride induced lipid peroxidation in the rat kidney. Toxicol Appl Pharmacol. Vol 73, No. 3:395-401, 1984.

Goodman and Gilman's The Pharmacological Basis of Therapeutics, Sixth Edition. Macmillan Publishing Co., Inc. NY, 1980.

Ha C. et al. The effect of vitamin B6 deficiency on cytotoxic immune responses of T cell, antibodies, and natural killer cells, and phagocytosis by macrophages. Cellular Immunology. Vol. 85:310-329, 1984.

Hendler S.S. The Doctors' Vitamin and Mineral Encyclopedia. Fireside Books, Simon & Schuster, New York, 1990.

Hill K.E. and Burk R.F. Influence of vitamin E and selenium on glutathione dependent protection against microsomal lipid peroxidation. Biochemical Pharmacology, Vol. 33, No.7:1065-1068, 1984.

Kosta L. et al. Correlation between selenium and mercury in man following exposure to inorganic mercury. Nature (London), Vol. 254:238-239, 1975.

Kutsky R.J. Handbook of Vitamins, Minerals and Hormones, Van Nostrand Reinhold Co., New York, 1981.

1984-85 Yearbook of Nutritional Medicine, Keats Publishing, Inc. New Canaan, CT. Edited by Jeffery Bland.

Masukawa R. et al. Differential changes of glutathione-S-transferase activity by dietary selenium. Biochemical Pharmacology, Vol 33, No.16:2635-2639, 1984.

Moeschlin S. (Ed), Klinik und Therapie der Vergiftungen. 6th edition. 1980. G. Threme, Verlag.

Nutrition Reviews' Present Knowledge in Nutrition (5th ed). The Nutrition Foundation, Inc. Washington, D.C. 1984.

Rowland I.R. et al. Effects of diet on mercury metabolism and excretion in mice given methylmercury: Role of gut flora. Archives of Environmental Health, Vol. 39, No. 6:401-408, 1984.

Sprince et al. Federation Proceedings, Vol. 33, No. 1, March, 1974.

Sturman J.A. et al. Effects of deficiency of vitamin B6 on transulfuration. Biochem Med. Vol. 3:244-251, 1969.

Tateishi N. et al. Journal of Nutrition, vol 112:2717-2226, 1982

Meister A. and Anderson M. Glutathione. Annual Reviews of Biochemistry, Vol 52:711-760, 1983.

Ziff S. and Ziff M.F. Dentistry Without Mercury, Bio-Probe,Inc Orlando, FL. 1993.

Ziff S. and Ziff M.F. Infertility and Birth Defects - Is Mercury From Silver Dental Fillings An Unsuspected Cause? Bio-Probe, Inc. Orlando, FL, 1987.

CHAPTER 15

THE MERCURY ISSUE UPDATED TO 1994

A great deal has happened since the 1986 revision, including ever increasing media attention.

Sweden continues to be in the forefront of doing something about stopping the use of amalgam. There have been a series of events, all publicized in newspapers, television, and government publications airing all the pro and con arguments. In 1987, the results of an eighteen month study by a government Expert Commission on the safety of amalgam were published. One of the conclusions reached was: "Amalgam is an unsuitable dental material from a toxicological point of view and should be banned as soon as a suitable replacement is available. In the interim, amalgam work in pregnant women should be kept to an absolute minimum." This same warning on the use of amalgam in pregnant women was also issued in Germany.

The issuance of the Expert Commission findings created further heated debate within the dental community and in the political arena. This led to some reorganization of responsibility with regard to mercury within the Swedish government. In early 1989, because of the fact that mercury is such a wide spread pollutant, responsibility for determining its overall environmental impact was transferred to the Chemical Inspection Directorate. In an October 6, 1989 press conference, Dr. Kerstin Niblaeus Director of the Chemical Inspection stated: ..."This week the Inspection sent the government a list of 10 hazardous chemicals which should be removed. On that list is mercury, a substance which is a component of amalgam. A ban on amalgam is a decision which the government must take, but Niblaeus is sure: I have not even considered that the government should not decide on a prohibition. ... The question is not if, but when we ban amalgam, Kerstin Niblaeus emphasizes. Mercury is not degraded in nature. Instead it accumulates and causes damage to animal and plant life. In addition it has been shown that amalgam can cause disease in humans."

Previously, on Sept 26, 1989, the Center Party Parliament Group had also issued a press release with the following heading: "NO AMALGAM AFTER 1991." The release went on to say: "The use of amalgam as a dental filling material must cease. Amalgam contains mercury. This is dissolved into the human body and causes physical and psychological damage. Alternative materials are already present. With intensified research there will be satisfactory materials in about a year. By stating a time limit for amalgam, developments will come faster. Therefore parliament should prohibit amalgam from 1992!"

On November 21, 1990, The Swedish Parliament decided that anyone who wants to exchange their amalgam fillings for alternative materials will be able to do so. The state will pay the costs according the dental insurance system, i.e., up to $500.00 the patient pays 60% of the cost, above $500.00 the patient pays 25% of the cost.

Special dental or medical examinations will no longer be necessary, nor will pre-approval from the insurance system be required before the exchange is started.

Finally, on 18 February 1994, the Swedish Government announced that amalgam will be totally banned for children and adolescents (up to 19 years of age) prior to 1 July 1995 and for the rest of the population not later than 1 January 1997. Several counties in Sweden have already stopped the use of amalgam in children and adolescents and the county of Blekinge has stopped the use of amalgam as a dental restorative material. The Swedish government will implement measures to increase knowledge of alternative materials and techniques both in the basic education and post graduate education of dental personnel.

Preceding the above announcement by the Swedish government was a dramatic (17 January 1994) public announcement on Stockholm TV by an officer of the Swedish Dental Association (SDA). Based on the results of a special meeting of the SDA held on 18 December 1993, the Chairman of the SDA Committee for Methodological and Quality Issues, announced a total reversal of their defense of the safety and use of dental amalgam, acknowledging that their leadership had previously been wrong on the subject.

The events in Germany regarding the amalgam controversy, have been almost as dramatic as those in Sweden. In 1987, the Federal

Department of Health (BGA) of the German government issued an advisory warning against the use of dental amalgam in pregnant women. On 2 February 1992, following an extraordinary Congress on dental amalgam sponsored by the International Academy of Oral Medicine and Toxicology (IAOMT), the BGA banned the manufacture and sale of low-copper conventional amalgam. Shortly thereafter, the BGA issued a document further restricting the use of amalgam, including the high-copper, non-gamma2-amalgam.

Then on 21 December 1993, Degussa AG, Germany's largest producer of dental amalgam announced that it would no longer provide the product. This was followed shortly thereafter, on 25 January 1994, by the public announcement by Professor Dr. Gustav Drasch of the Institute of Forensic Medicine of the University of Munich, revealing the results of a recent research study. The study measured the mercury content of the kidneys, liver and brain tissue of deceased fetuses, newborn and young children. The mercury levels correlated directly to the amount of dental amalgam in the teeth of the mothers. These results clearly demonstrated that the mercury from the dental amalgams of mothers is inherited by their offspring. It confirmed previous findings in animal studies reported by scientists at the University of Calgary, Canada. The German BGA immediately repeated their warning that pregnant women and women of child bearing age should avoid dental amalgam treatments.

Meanwhile here in the United States, the American Dental Association (ADA), was taking a most unusual step. In June 1987, the ADA amended their "Principles of Ethics and Code of Professional Conduct: to make it improper and unethical for any ADA dentist to recommend or suggest removal of amalgam fillings, from the nonallergic patient, for the alleged purpose of removing toxic substances from the body. To the best of my knowledge, this is the first time in the history of the ADA that a dental material has been singled out for such special treatment. In effect, it is a warning to all dentists not to say or imply anything to any patient about mercury or any of its potential harmful effects.

Although we talked about the ADA patient pamphlet on Dental Amalgam in Chapter 4, I failed to bring out a very serious error. The untruth contained in the ADA Brochure W186 reads "More than 50 years ago, the American Dental Association established a certification program to help dentists choose from among the safest and most effective of these brands. Currently more than 100 brands of amalgam have been certified for dentists' use." However, in a letter dated May 22, 1986, the ADA stated: "The amalgam does not form until the dentist mixes the alloy with mercury. Therefore, dental amalgam per se cannot be certified. We cannot certify a reaction product made by the dentist."

The same philosophy was in evidence when the Food and Drug Administration's Final Rule on Dental Devices was published in the Federal Register of August 12, 1987. After 10 years of drafting the Final Rule, the whole issue of classifying amalgam as a dental device was neatly avoided by only classifying mercury and the dental alloy with which it is mixed to make amalgam. By saying that they were only classifying the components of amalgam and not the amalgam itself, which must be mixed in the dental office, the FDA Dental Devices Panel was able to circumvent the more stringent controls imposed by the FDA on implants. As amalgam was not being classified there was no need to consider it as an implant. As an implant, amalgam would have to be proven biocompatible, before the FDA could approve its use in humans.

It is interesting to note that the dental device panel established by the FDA to do the evaluation did not have a single member who was a toxicologist, physiologist, allergist/dermatologist, or physician. The potential health hazards of mercury and amalgam dental fillings were evaluated and approved by personnel who had no medical qualifications to do so. Meanwhile, scientists and medical researchers all over the world have been diligently working to unravel the mystery of mercury toxicity associated with amalgam fillings.

Further validation of the 1984 and 1986 brain autopsy studies was achieved with publication, in 1987, of a major study by David Eggleston, DDS (Associate Professor, USC School of Dentistry) and Magnus Nylander DDS (Karolinska Institute in Sweden). Brain autopsy studies, conducted on 77 cadavers of accidental death, replicated the German and Swedish studies confirming the correlation between brain mercury levels and the numbers and surfaces of amalgam dental fillings. Their work demonstrated that individuals with amalgam fillings had about three times more mercury in their brain than people without amalgam fillings.

Also in 1987, Nylander, Friberg and Lind published the results of a 34 person autopsy study again confirming the association between amalgam load and accumulation of mercury in tissues. This study also demonstrated that amalgam bearers had significantly higher mercury levels in the kidney cortex than did amalgam-free individuals.

With regard to brain mercury levels, work being done at the University of Kentucky on the possible causes of Alzheimer's disease is very exciting. Autopsy studies done on 180 individuals who had died during 1985-1990 of Alzheimer's disease has revealed striking elevations of mercury in specific areas of the brain involved in Alzheimer's disease. Unfortunately, dental status and dental histories were not collected or investigated. Therefore, it will remain a mystery whether the high mercury levels found were related to the numbers and surfaces of amalgam fillings these individuals dying of Alzheimer's disease might have had. Although there is no way of knowing for sure, it would seem logical to assume that the only common or universal mercury exposure that this diverse geographical group of Kentuckians could have had was their mercury dental fillings. Funding for a follow-on five year study of Alzheimer's disease and its possible relationship to dental amalgam has been obtained and is being conducted by Dr. William Markesbery and his group at the University of Kentucky Sanders-Brown Center on Aging.

Other research studies at the University of Kentucky are producing further dramatic evidence connecting mercury as a probable etiological factor in the development of Alzheimer's disease. At the 75th annual meeting of the Federation of American Societies for Experiment Biology (FASEB), E. Duhr and his associates presented the results of their animal study demonstrating that mercury caused the same reaction in brain GTP-tubulin as that seen in Alzheimer's disease brain samples. Their conclusion was "These results suggest that certain complexed forms of Hg^{2+} must be considered as a potential source for the etiology of Alzheimer's disease." In the same study, administration of aluminum failed to cause the Alzheimer's type damage.

The text book "Biological Monitoring of Toxic Metals" was published in 1988. The book contains a chapter titled "The prediction of intake of mercury vapor from amalgams" which was written by Dr. Lars Friberg and Dr. Thomas W. Clarkson, two of the foremost mercury toxicologists in the world. The following six major points represent the conclusions drawn from their investigations:

1. The evidence indicates that amalgam surfaces release mercury vapor into the mouth.

2. The rate of release is increased by stressing the amalgam surface by chewing and brushing.

3. The surface layer does not immediately repair after stress and that it may take several hours to completely restore the surface layer.

4. The release of mercury from amalgam results in the deposition of mercury in body tissue and an increase in urinary excretion.

5. The estimated release rates from amalgam appear to be consistent with levels of mercury found in autopsy tissue in the general population and with increases in brain and urinary levels due to amalgam fillings.

6. The release of mercury from dental amalgams makes the predominant contribution to human exposure to inorganic mercury including mercury vapor in the general population.

The publication of this data by these world renowned researchers was of great significance in validating and adding to the existing bench mark data on the release and deposition of mercury from amalgam.

In 1988 the University of Calgary Medical School embarked on a series of research investigations into the release, distribution, and possible pathology of mercury from dental fillings. The initial studies were undertaken using sheep as the research animal. Amalgam fillings containing a portion of radioactively labelled elemental mercury were placed in 12 molar teeth. Extreme care was taken in the placement of these fillings - i.e., one-half the normal amount of amalgam utilized in occlusal fillings in humans was utilized; the biting surface of the completed fillings were concave by design, eliminating direct contact between opposing fillings; the throat was packed and the oral cavity was flushed and rinsed several times to insure that no residual mercury resulting from the placement of the fillings remained in the oral cavity.

The first paper was published in 1989 and demonstrated that mercury will appear in various organs and tissues within 29 days.

There were three uptake sites: lung, gastrointestinal, and jaw tissue absorption. Once absorbed, high concentrations of dental amalgam mercury rapidly localized in the kidneys and liver. The data also showed mercury accumulation from dental amalgams in the brain, pituitary, thyroid, adrenal, pancreas, and ovary.

In 1990 the next paper of the Calgary group outlined the results of their study showing the maternal-fetal distribution of radioactive mercury released from dental amalgam fillings that had been placed in pregnant sheep. This study demonstrated that mercury from dental amalgam will appear in maternal blood, fetal blood, and amniotic fluid within two days after placement of amalgam fillings. Maternal concentrations of amalgam mercury were highest in the kidneys and liver. In the fetus the highest concentrations of amalgam mercury appeared in the liver and pituitary gland. This study also demonstrated that the milk concentration of amalgam mercury postpartum provides a potential source of mercury exposure to newborn. The authors concluded: "In view of the experimental evidence presented herein, continued employment of dental amalgam as a tooth restorative material in pregnant women and children should be reconsidered."

It is apparent that mercury investigative scientists, researchers and toxicologists all over the world share a common concern about exposing pregnant women and children to mercury, from any source. All of which presents a real dilemma for women who are pregnant and women who are nursing their babies. Should they have their amalgam fillings replaced during pregnancy or during nursing? There is no scientific research to support an answer one way or the other. Scientists have not measured the increase in total body burden of mercury during the nine months of pregnancy compared to the increase in body burden that might result from full mouth replacement of amalgam fillings. The same is true for nursing mothers. The animal data shows that mothers' milk contains four times more mercury than in the mothers' blood. However, here again, there is no scientific data measuring the variation of mercury in mothers' milk before, during, and after amalgam replacement. The warning to pregnant women issued in Sweden and Germany should be taken seriously, i.e, if at all possible, avoid any dental work involving mercury amalgam during pregnancy. All dental work should be kept to an absolute minimum during pregnancy. Do not get your amalgam fillings polished and do not chew gum.

In October of 1990, two abstracts showing pathology directly related to dental amalgam mercury were presented at the annual meeting of the American Physiology Association. The first abstract from the University of Calgary Medical School provided the results of a research experiment in which amalgam fillings were placed in six adult female sheep. Kidney function was evaluated several days prior to amalgam placement and 30 and 60 days after placement. Within 60 days there was almost a 50% impairment of kidney function. The full study was subsequently published in the American Journal of Physiology in 1991.

In the second abstract, from the University of Georgia Microbiology Department by A.O. Summers and J. Wireman, fecal and gingival microbial flora samples were taken from two adult monkeys in which amalgam fillings had been placed (University of Calgary). Mercury resistance in gingival and fecal flora began occurring 10 days after amalgam placement. Mercury resistant means that these bacteria convert inorganic and organic mercury (which would normally be excreted in the feces) to volatile, lipid soluble mercury vapor, which is then recycled back into the blood. This same family of bacteria are also present in humans. Dr. Summers believes that these bacteria carry in their genetic material resistance to several commonly used antibiotic drugs. Further, there appears to be a growing drug resistance in bacteria which is seriously limiting options in fighting infectious diseases.

Dr. Summers final paper on mercury resistant and antibiotic resistant bacteria was published in 1993. This is a major breakthrough study addressing what is becoming one of the most important issues in modern medicine, i.e. the development of antibiotic resistance in major segments of the populations around the world. The seriousness of the situation was recently addressed in a major article appearing in the March 28, 1994 issue of Newsweek, which carried the heading of "The End of Antibiotics." Unfortunately, the authors of the article were not aware of the mercury resistant aspect of the problem. However, the 1993 paper by Dr. Summers and her associates clearly demonstrated, in animal studies, that the antibiotic resistance disappeared when the source of mercury was removed.

These studies demonstrating pathology were immediately attacked by the ADA as being flawed and for using sheep, which the ADA claims are a poor animal upon which to do human research. This same diatribe was reiterated by the spokesman for the FDA Dental Devices section.

The fact that mercury from amalgam dental fillings had the potential of causing pathological damage in humans triggered an onslaught of major media attention: Chicago Tribune, Aug 15, 1990, 5 col front page article; Insight Oct 1, 1990, a full page article; USA Today, October 9, 1990, front page article; Newsweek, October 15, 1990, a 3 col full page article; USA Today, October 24, 1990, a full half-page article; San Jose Mercury News (San Jose, California) Nov 15, 1990, front page article; New York Times, Dec 13, 1990, a four column spread across the top of the Health section. There were major articles in at least 20 other newspapers and magazines that I am personally aware of and the actual number is probably somewhere between 40-100. In addition, radio talk-shows and news programs carried the story to hundreds of other communities.

The peak of all this activity occurred on December 16, 1990, when the award winning CBS program 60-Minutes took a double segment of the show to air a major investigative report on the amalgam controversy. The name of the report was "Is there a poison in your mouth?" The program presented an impartial, objective, in-depth look at all sides of the amalgam issue and, according to information from CBS, they received more calls, letters, requests for transcripts and video tapes than any previous program.

It would not be unreasonable to estimate that in the last three months of 1990, more than fifty million people in the United States and Canada were exposed to the following facts:

- » Silver dental fillings, that most people in industrialized countries have in their teeth, contain 45-50% mercury.
- » Mercury is a heavy poisonous metal, more toxic than lead or arsenic.
- » The mercury continuously released by these fillings has the potential of causing serious health problems.

In 1990 two additional studies demonstrating the distribution of mercury from amalgam dental fillings were published. Both of these studies used monkeys as the research animal. (The medical and scientific research communities have accepted the results of monkey research as closely paralleling that which might be expected in humans). Danscher and colleagues in Denmark published the results of a one year study in monkeys with amalgam dental fillings and Vimy and associates in Canada published the results of their monkey study. Both studies demonstrated similar distribution patterns for mercury from amalgam fillings and also provided confirmation of the distribution patterns that had been found in the sheep studies. Mercury from dental amalgam fillings was found in the brain and in every gland and organ.

In early 1991, the ADA expended a tremendous amount of money and effort in damage-control in an attempt to overcome the effects of the unprecedented nationwide media attention. ADA headquarters and ADA dentists were being deluged with calls questioning the safety of their silver amalgam dental fillings. The ADA provided every dentist in the United States with information: Statements from government agencies, heads of biomaterial departments in dental schools, Deans of dental schools, the President of the ADA, foreign scientists and the Canadian Dental Association, all testifying to the safety of dental amalgam; a list of scientific studies that they felt supported the safety of dental amalgam.

Two of the studies held up as proving that amalgam is safe were epidemiology studies done in Sweden. The first study was published in 1988 by Ahlqwist and associates and an extension of this study was published in 1989 by Lavstedt and Sundberg. Unfortunately, both studies arrived at their conclusions by comparing people with amalgams to other people with a fewer number of amalgams. Neither study compared amalgam bearers to people who had never had amalgam fillings. Health status was determined by an unsupervised, self-administered questionnaire of symptom complaints. It should also be noted that any neurological pathology, well established to be attributable to mercury exposure, was not requested or reported. The quality of the studies were such, that it is doubtful that either study would have been accepted for publication in a peer reviewed medical journal.

This same public relations blitz contained information that

questioned the validity of the study methodology and the results obtained from the studies done at the University of Calgary. The ADA also modified its interpretation of the ethics ruling prohibiting replacement of amalgam fillings. The new interpretation permits the dentist to replace amalgam fillings and to talk about mercury amalgam if requested by the patient. However, the ADA dentist is still restricted from talking about the mercury controversy or recommending or suggesting replacement of amalgam fillings with a non-mercury filling or restoration.

On March 15, 1991, the FDA Dental Products Panel of the Medical Devices Advisory Committee met to hear testimony on whether to classify dental amalgam as a Class III dental device. Placement in Class III would have required the manufacturers to prove the safety of amalgam.

After a full day of testimony from various speakers, the Panel voted unanimously on two resolutions: 1. Insufficient evidence was presented to justify classifying amalgam as unsafe but questions were raised that require scientific investigation. 2. A committee should be formed to define the required areas of investigation and the appropriate research to resolve the question of amalgam safety.

The latter is certainly a worthwhile objective. However, there is a serious problem with the actions of the panel, both past and present. To wit: The Medical Device Amendment to the Federal Food, Drug, and Cosmetic Act signed into law on 28 May 1976 requires the FDA to classify all medical (including dental) devices "intended for human use" in the United States. If a material is not classified under the law it cannot be considered an approved dental device.

Herein lies the real problem and miscarriage of Congressional intent. The Final Rule of the FDA on Classification of Dental Devices was published in the Federal Register on 12 August 1987. There is no mention in this document of dental amalgam as a dental device. To avoid the issue of classifying amalgam, the FDA accepted and classified only the components of amalgam, i.e., dental mercury and amalgam alloy. The acceptance and classification of these two components without ever classifying the final product that results when the two components are mixed into "amalgam" and implanted in the patients teeth, is a clear violation of the law and the FDA rules mandating that classified medical devices must be both safe and effective.

Neither component of amalgam can be used alone as a dental device. Dental mercury (which is elemental mercury) cannot be used by itself as a dental filling material. The same is true for amalgam alloy. If either of these two components were to be placed in a tooth prepared for filling, without first being mixed together, they would rapidly wash out. Therefore, both materials fail the FDA rule requirement for "EFFECTIVENESS". The Dental Device Panel erred in classifying them in the first place, and the FDA is obligated to correct that error by withdrawing their classification.

A very recent letter (subsequent to the March 15, 1991 meeting of the Dental Products Panel) from the FDA, Director, Division of Ob-Gyn, ENT, and Dental Devices, Office of Device Evaluation states in part "I must remind you that FDA regulates manufacturers of medical devices. No manufacturer produces mixed dental amalgams. The mixed dental amalgam is prepared by dental clinicians. FDA does regulate manufacturers of dental mercury and amalgam alloys, but the only control FDA has over the ultimate, mixed amalgam is through the labeling for dental mercury and amalgam alloys. The Federal Food, Drug, and Cosmetic Act does not empower FDA to regulate the manner in which dental clinicians mix dental mercury and amalgam alloys to make dental amalgams."

The above actions by the Federal Agency charged with responsibility to protect the public from the use of unsafe dental devices, and the ADA, the largest U.S. trade organization representing the dental profession, have placed the dental clinician in the untenable position of being a manufacturer of dental amalgam. Therefore, every dentist in the United States who implants a dental amalgam filling in a patient's tooth, is in violation of the Federal Rules and Regulations governing the manufacture of implants and dental devices. Each dentist who wishes to "manufacture" dental amalgam must apply to the Federal Government for approval of the implant device. In order to secure FDA approval, the manufacturer must provide sufficient scientific evidence to the Dental Products Panel, FDA Office of Device Evaluation, so that the proper classification of the device may be made and a rule for its use established.

Two of the presenters at the March 15, 1991 FDA meeting were Dr. Lars Friberg and Dr. Thomas W. Clarkson, both of whom presented data that is contained in the revision of the World Health Organization (WHO) criteria document on exposure to inorganic mercury. Of particular interest were the WHO conclusions regarding the estimated intake of mercury from all sources:

Dental amalgam fillings = 3.0-17.5 micrograms per day (mercury vapor);
fish = 2.4 micrograms per day (methylmercury);
non-fish food = 0.3 micrograms per day (inorganic mercury).
Other sources including air and water were found to be negligible.

The magnitude of amalgam related mercury body burden has subsequently been confirmed by Professor H. Vasken Aposhian and his colleagues at the University of Arizona. Their 1992 study demonstrated that two-thirds of the mercury excreted in the urine of those with dental amalgams was derived originally from the mercury vapor released from their amalgams. Dr. Aposhian's work confirmed the results of a 1992 study by Dr. Zander and his associates in Germany, who concluded that the release of mercury from amalgam fillings represented the main source of mercury exposure in subjects with amalgam fillings.

The conclusions of the WHO committee on mercury, and those of Dr's Aposhian and Zander, are in sharp variance with those of the ADA and other pro-mercury advocates, who all claim that patient intake of mercury from amalgam dental fillings is minimal when compared to the average intake from fish. One possible reason for the difference in conclusions is that the researchers involved in the Arizona and Germany studies and the WHO committee on mercury, which was comprised of world class scientists, did not have a pro or con-amalgam agenda. Their primary concern was an objective evaluation of the scientific data and a presentation of their conclusions.

In January 1993 the Public Health Service published their report on the safety of amalgam which had taken twenty-five months to write. The Preface of the Final Report sums up the veracity of the entire effort: "This report is not intended to serve as the authoritative source on dental amalgam safety, but rather as a planning tool to assist policy-makers in deciding on appropriate risk management actions."

One the conclusions of the report was "Available data are not sufficient to indicate that health hazards can be identified in non-occupationally exposed persons. Health hazards, however, cannot be dismissed." Throughout the report their are caveats of the same nature, indicating insufficient data was available to make sound pronouncements about human health risks from dental amalgam.

Unfortunately, these findings had no bearing on the Press Release put out by the Public Health Service which was designed to assure the U.S. population that there is no solid evidence of any harm for millions of Americans who have amalgam fillings and that there is no persuasive reason to avoid amalgams or any necessity to have them removed.

In October 1987, the Foundation For Toxic Free Dentistry (FTFD) was chartered in the state of Florida. FTFD is a 501(c)(3) non-profit tax-exempt organization. One of the primary purposes of the Foundation is to disseminate information regarding the amalgam issue that reflects what is contained in the scientific literature. Another major purpose of FTFD is to maintain a listing of mercury-free dentists. FTFD provides referrals to any individual making the decision to have all further dental work performed by a professional who is aware of the scientific literature and understands the dangers of unnecessarily exposing a patient to mercury vapor. Further, mercury-free dentists, are usually more experienced in the proper placement of alternative materials, which are very technique sensitive.

Since its inception in 1987 the Foundation had received hundreds of letters from individuals describing how the simple act of removing mercury from their teeth had ameliorated or cured various health conditions of long standing. The problem with all this correspondence was that it was coming to the Foundation and not to the FDA, who really needed to be made aware of the magnitude of the amalgam health problem. Consequently, in early 1991, the FTFD developed the Patient's Adverse Reaction Report, which was a simple form on which the patient could list symptoms and indicate whether they got better, worse, or did not change after amalgam replacement. The original of the form was to be sent to the FDA and the 2nd copy was to be returned to the FTFD.

The results of over 700 reports submitted to the FDA were very dramatic. During the same period, several other studies reflecting the changes in symptomatology after amalgam replacement were being performed in Canada, Sweden, Denmark, and the United States. The results of these studies demonstrated that in the vast majority of individuals who have undergone amalgam replacement and the subsequent reduction of their mercury body burden, there were improvements in health that have ranged from minor to startlingly dramatic. For example the statistics listed below were compiled by the FTFD on 1569 patients from 6 different reports:

% of Total	SYMPTOM	Total No. No.	Improved or Cured	% of cure or Improvement
14%	ALLERGY	221	196	89%
5%	ANXIETY	86	80	93%
5%	BAD TEMPER	81	68	89%
6%	BLOATING	88	70	88%
6%	BLOOD PRESSURE PROBLEMS	99	53	54%
5%	CHEST PAINS	79	69	87%
22%	DEPRESSION	347	315	91%
22%	DIZZINESS	343	301	88%
45%	FATIGUE	705	603	86%
15%	GASTROINTESTINAL PROBLEMS	231	192	83%
8%	GUM PROBLEMS	129	121	94%
34%	HEADACHES	531	460	87%
3%	MIGRAINE HEADACHES	45	39	87%
12%	INSOMNIA	187	146	78%
10%	IRREGULAR HEARTBEAT	159	139	87%
8%	IRRITABILITY	132	119	90%
17%	LACK OF CONCENTRATION	270	216	80%
6%	LACK OF ENERGY	91	88	97%
17%	MEMORY LOSS	265	193	73%
17%	METALLIC TASTE	260	247	95%
7%	MULTIPLE SCLEROSIS	113	86	76%
8%	MUSCLE TREMOR	126	104	83%
10%	NERVOUSNESS	158	131	83%

8% NUMBNESS ANYWHERE	118	97	82%
20% SKIN DISTURBANCES	310	251	81%
9% SORE THROAT	149	128	86%
6% TACHYCARDIA	97	68	70%
4% THYROID PROBLEMS	56	44	79%
12% ULCERS & SORES (ORAL CAVITY)	189	162	86%
7% URINARY TRACT PROBLEMS	115	87	76%
29% VISION PROBLEMS	462	289	63%

The above statistics involve a total of 1569 patients in different studies: 762 patients utilized the FTFD Patient Adverse Reaction Report to individually report changes in their health directly to the FDA and the FTFD; Dr.Mats Hanson, Ph.D. reported on 519 Swedish patients; Henrik Lichtenberg, D.D.S. of Denmark reported on 100 patients; Pierre LaRose, D.D.S. of Canada reported on 80 patients; Robert L.Siblerud O.D., M.S. reported on 86 patients in Colorado as partial fulfillment of a Ph.D.requirement; and Albert V.Zamm, M.D., FACA, FACP reported on 22 of his patients.

One extremely interesting statistic relates to the incidence of allergies. The recent January 1993 Public Health Service Report on Dental Amalgam states that the incidence of allergic reaction to amalgam dental fillings is extremely rare, with only 50 case histories being reported in the literature. Statements of this nature totally ignore valid peer reviewed scientific studies demonstrating an allergic reaction to dental amalgam ranging from 16.5% for non-allergic patients to 44% for fourth year dental students. More importantly, as this symptom analysis demonstrates, the question is not whether the patient is allergic to dental amalgam but rather the direct causal relationship of mercury/amalgam dental fillings to the development of allergies to food, chemicals, and environmental factors.

In the FTFD analysis, this is supported by the fact that 14% of the individuals reported some type of allergy and that after replacement of their mercury/amalgam dental fillings, 89% reported their condition had improved or was totally eliminated. If you were to extrapolate this data to the approximately 140 million amalgam bearers in the United States, there should be 19.6 million people (14%) with amalgam causally related allergies. Of this number 89%

or approximately 17.4 million would have their allergies ameliorate or disappear simply by having their mercury dental fillings exchanged for non-mercury ones.

We attempted to look at this from another perspective by first determining the total number of people in the U.S. with allergies. Although there are no hard data available, the NIH estimates the number to be between 40-50 million. Using the lesser number of 40 million people with allergies, it is estimated that 65% or 26 million of them would be amalgam bearers whose allergies may be causally related to their mercury/amalgam dental fillings.

One last thought - throughout all of these years of the ADA and FDA denial and denigration of the scientific research, there have been thousands of case histories of people from all over the world who have had cures or some degree of health improvement in intractable medical problems simply through the removal and replacement of amalgam fillings with non-mercury materials. How long can this overwhelming clinical evidence be ignored or dismissed?

REFERENCES

Aposhian HV et al. Urinary mercury after administration of 2,3-dimercaptopropane-1sulfonic acid: correlation with dental score. FASEB J. 6(6):2472-2476, April 1992.

Ahlqwist M. et al. Number of amalgam tooth fillings in relation to subjectively experienced symptoms in a study of Swedish women. Commun Dent Oral Epidemiol. 16:227-231, 1988.

Boyd ND, Benediktsson H, Vimy MJ, Hooper DE, and Lorscheider FL. Mercury from dental "silver" tooth fillings impairs sheep kidney function. Am J Physiol. 261 (Regulatory Integrative Comp. Physiol. 30): R1010-R1014, 1991.

Clarkson TW, Friberg L, Nordberg GF, and Sager PR.(Editors) Biological Monitoring of Toxic Metals, pp 247-264, Plenum Press NY, 1988.

Danscher G, Horsted-Bindslev P, and Rungby J.Traces of mercury in organs from primates with amalgam fillings. Exp Molecular Pathol. 52:291-299, 1990.

DENTAL AMALGAM: A scientific review and recommended Public Health Service strategy for research, education and regulation.January 1993, Department of Health and Human Services, Public Health Service, Washington, D.C.

Duhr E, Pendergrass C, Kasarskis E, Slevin J, and Haley B.Hg2+ induces gtp-tubulin interactions in rat brain similar to those observed in Alzheimer's disease.FASEB, 75th Annual Meeting, Atlanta,GA April 21-25, 1991 Abstract #493.

Eggleston DW and Nylander, M. Correlation of dental amalgam with mercury in brain tissue. Journal of Prosthetic Dentistry, Vol 58, No 6, Dec 1987.

Federal Register Wed.Aug.12, 1987, Part VI Dept.of Health and Human Services, Food and Drug Administration; 21 CFR Part 872. Medical Devices; Dental Devices Classification; Final Rule and Withdrawal of Proposed Rules.Volume 52, No.155, pages 30082 - 30108.

Hahn LJ, Kloiber R, Leininger RW, Vimy MJ, and Lorscheider FL. Whole-body imaging of the distribution of mercury released from dental fillings into monkey tissues.FASEB J.4:3256-3260, Nov 1990.

Hahn LJ, Kloiber R, Vimy MJ, Takahashi Y, and Lorscheider FL. Dental "silver" tooth fillings: a source of mercury exposure revealed by whole-body image scan and tissue analysis.FASEB J.3:2641-2646; Dec.1989.

Health fillings should stay put, ADA council says.ADA News, Sept 7, 1987.

Lavstedt S. and Sundberg H. Medical diagnoses and symptom related to amalgam fillings. TandLäkartidn. 84:81-88, 1989.

Nylander M., Friberg L., and Lind B. Mercury concentrations in the human brain and kidneys in relation to exposure from dental amalgam fillings. Swed Dent J.11:179-187, 1987.

Summers AO, and Wireman J. Increased mercury resistance in monkey gingival and intestinal bacterial flora after placement of dental silver fillings. The Physiologist 33(4), A-116, Aug 1990.

Summers AO, Wireman J, Vimy MJ, Lorscheider FL, Marshall B, Levy SB, Bennett S, and Billard L. Mercury released from dental "silver" fillings provokes an increase in mercury and antibiotic resistant bacteria in the primate oral and intestinal flora. Antimicrobial Agents & Chemotherapy.Vol 37:825-834, 1993.

The Alzheimer's Disease Research Center Update Newsletter, Fall 1991, University of Kentucky, Lexington, Kentucky.

Vimy MJ, Boyd ND, Hooper DE and Lorscheider FL. Glomerular filtration impairment by mercury released from dental "silver" fillings in sheep. The Physiologist 33(4), A-94, Aug 1990.

Vimy MJ, Takahashi Y, and Lorscheider FL. Maternal-fetal distribution of mercury (203Hg) released from dental amalgam fillings.American Journal of Physiology 258 (Regulatory Integrative Comp.Physiol.27):R939-R945, 1990.

Jim Warren. Alzheimer's may be linked to mercury, University of Kentucky scientists say. Lexington Herald-Leader, October 17, 1990.

World Health Organization, Environmental Health Criteria 118, Geneva, 1991.

Zander D,. et al. Studies on human exposure to mercury. 3. DMPS induced mobilization of mercury in subjects with and without amalgam fillings. Zentralblatt fur Hygiene und Umwelmedizin. 192(5):447-454, Feb 1992.

Zamm AV. Removal of dental mercury: Often an effective treatment for the very sensitive patient. J Orthomol Med 5(3):138-142, 1990.

Ziff S.and Ziff MF. Dental Mercury - An Environmental Hazard! Bio-Probe Newsletter 8(5):1-6, Sept 1992.

For a complete catalog write:

AURORA PRESS
P.O. BOX 573
SANTA FE NEW MEXICO 87504

TMJ - THE JAW CONNECTION
THE OVERLOOKED DIAGNOSIS

A SELF-CARE GUIDE TO DIAGNOSING AND MANAGING THIS HIDDEN AILMENT

Greg Goddard, D.D.S.

"It is estimated that 28 percent of the U.S. population hasTMJ."
Public Citizen *Health Letter*

"This is an excellent comprehensive guide to TMJ. I highly recommend it to patients."
C. Norman Shealy, M.D., Ph.D.

A comprehensive guide empowering TMJ sufferers to uncover and treat this prevalent, often misdiagnosed ailment that plagues an estimated fifty million Americans. Many of us have TMJ (Temporomandibular Joint) disorders without knowing it. Several seemingly unrelated conditions may indicate a jaw dysfunction. For instance, do you suffer from one or more of the following?

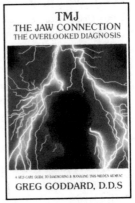

* Jaw fatigue upon awakening from sleep
* Unexplained headaches
* Unexplained pain in or above the ears
* Clicking or popping of the jaw
* Grinding or clenching of teeth
* Ringing or hissing in the ears
* Deviation of jaw movement when opening the mouth
* Excessive wearing down of the teeth
* Unexplained dizziness

These and other signs should alert you that you may be pursuing a cure for a misdiagnosed condition that could be costing unnecessary time and expense as well as unwarranted medical tests and/or dental work.

The author, Dr. Greg Goddard, combines his extensive personal clinical experience with adjunctive therapies to help readers arrive at a treatment fitting their own circumstances. The role of muscles, joints, stress, tension, accidents, nutrition, dentistry and posture are among some of the topics explored.

ISBN: 0-943358-35-3 Paper 200 Pages 5&1/4 x 8&1/4

PULSE DIAGNOSIS

Detailed Interpretations For Eastern & Western Holistic Treatments

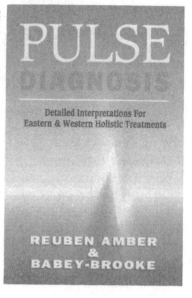

REUBEN AMBER

The most significant diagnostic technique available to the medical profession has always been the pulse. This unprecedented text presents a detailed examination of the possible interpretations of this simple indication of the presence of life, from the point of view of four major medical traditions. Included is the historical background, detailed analysis and descriptions of the diagnostic uses of the pulse in Iran, China, India and the West.

- Chinese Healing Precepts
- Ayurvedic Philosophy & The Pulse
- Technique Of Taking The Pulse
- Dreams & The Pulse
- The Pregnancy Pulse
- The Pulse & Organ Relationships
- Arabian Medicine & The Pulse
- Diseases & The Pulse
- Seasons & The Pulse
- The Death Pulse

Pulse Diagnosis is an unparalleled synthesis bridging the gap between contemporary scientific models and the Holistic approach integrating body, mind and spirit in the diagnosis. Dr. Amber offers a treasury of profound insights for all people in the healing professions.

ISBN:0-943358-41-8 Paperback 232 Pages 6x9 $14.95

THE EAR: GATEWAY TO BALANCING THE BODY

A MODERN GUIDE TO EAR ACUPUNCTURE

Mario Wexu, D.AC

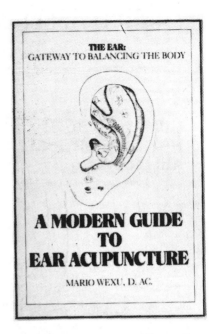

This is the first comprehensive modern textbook of ear acupuncture. The author uniquely combines his extensive personal clinical experience with traditional and modern Chinese and European sources. Anatomical descriptions with detailed charts clearly illustrate how to locate and use over three hundred ear points, both alone and in combination with body points, to treat and prevent illness. Case histories with specific techniques cover problems such as:

- Deafness
- Otitis
- Otalgia
- Drug Addiction
- Tobacco Addiction
- Alcoholism
- Obesity
- Anesthesia
- Oedema
- Insomnia
- Acupuncture Anesthesia
- Electronic Acupuncture Devices

An excellent repertory listing 130 diseases facilitates an understanding of this incredible and valuable healing art.

ISBN: 0-943358-08-6   **Paperback**   **6 × 9**   **217 Pages**   **$12.50**

WHY FLYING ENDANGERS YOUR HEALTH

**HIDDEN HEALTH
HAZARDS OF
AIR TRAVEL**

F. S. Kahn

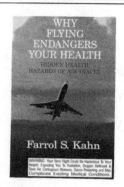

This uncompromising, hard-hitting expose of air travel opens our eyes for the first time to the serious health risks of flying and will change forever the way people think about air travel.

Is flying really safe? Why has so little been disclosed about the health hazards of flying? Are there some people who should not fly at all? The flying public has been kept in the dark too long about the health dangers of flying. F. S. Kahn reveals the technical causes of health dangers and gives concrete advice on how to avoid these risks.

Two invaluable checklists are provided: one for all passengers; one for high risk health conditions - which will enable you to make informed decisions about whether or not you should fly. Recommendations are given to help alleviate the health stressors routinely encountered in flight.

This book is compelling reading for all people who fly and in addition provides previously unavailable information for doctors, psychiatrists, and flight crews.

". . .this is the first time I have seen such comprehensive coverage in a commercially published book."
- New Scientist

". . .a controversial health warning to the globe trotting set."
-The Times

ISBN: 0-943358-36-1 Paper 305 Pages 5&1/4 x 8&1/4 $14.00